Addiction Medicine for Health Care Professionals

Addiction Medicine for Health Care Professionals

ROBERT D. LOVINGER, MD

ELSEVIER

Publisher: Cathleen Sether
Acquisition Editor: Joslyn Chaiprasert-Paguio
Editorial Project Manager: Rebeka Henry
Production Project Manager: Poulouse Joseph
Cover Designer: Miles Hitchen

3251 Riverport Lane
St. Louis, Missouri 63043

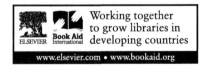

Working together
to grow libraries in
developing countries

www.elsevier.com • www.bookaid.org

*To my beloved wife Debra, children Rachel and Ashley,
and granddaughter Jade who have brought meaning to my life.*

*To my mentors, Drs. William Ganong, Selna Kaplan, Melvin Grumbach,
and Hanns Gruemer who introduced me to the joys of endocrinology, neurophysiology,
neuroscience, neurochemistry, and clinical chemistry.*

*To my dear friends Dr. David Loucas, an internist, and Dr. William Romanos,
a psychiatrist, who are now in a different and peaceful place in the universe,
whose dedication and passion to those suffering from substance abuse
disorders are an inspiration to me every day.*

Preface

This monograph is a labor of love and necessity. The love is derived from my interactions with my cherished patients who are and have been categorically underserved and in desperate need of help with their addictions, health (both physical and mental), and previously unable to find peace and enjoyment in their lives. During my extensive medical career, I feel honored and privileged to have had the opportunity to serve and provide these individuals with the support and hope for a better life in the future.

As a teacher throughout most of my career, I was fortunate to learn the basic principles of neurophysiology, neurochemistry, clinical chemistry, and compassionate clinical care early as a physician. As I became more involved in addiction medicine, I began to realize the understandable knowledge gaps, lack of mutual comprehension between medical and therapy services, and deficiency of uniformity in protocol standardization in my treatment provider colleagues (physicians, nurses, PA's, mental health counselors/ therapists, etc.) who were minimally or incompletely taught all these necessary specifics of this area of medicine throughout their entire training experience but were now trying to care for this difficult and complex patient group without all of the necessary "tools" at their fingertips, which could affect accurate and meaningful clinical decision-making.

Between the constant questions and discussions (often repeat) with my colleagues, students, residents, fellows, nurses, nurse practitioners, physician's assistants, therapists, and other healthcare professionals, both still in training or after its completion, over the years concerning these knowledge voids, it slowly became apparent to the author to try to help them in a more inclusive and insightful way, by writing a manuscript discussing the areas of this medical field that most of the questions were about. Thus, the reason for writing this book was to produce a more concise, comprehensive, understandable, and critical information-filled handbook, divided into five specific sections, based on the current medical literature and the authors extensive experience, which could quickly and easily provide the inquiring healthcare team member with the necessary information being sought in a precise, compact, easy-to-read and quick-find format spanning the essential nonmental health management side of substance abuse patient treatment.

This manuscript will hopefully bridge the gap, so needed information can now be easily obtained and reviewed when needed, as team members often have little time to search for, find, and read this information in one of the large, protracted, academically oriented, addiction medicine textbooks.

In addition, it is written to help addiction medicine professionals (physicians, nurses, physician's assistants, mental health clinicians, psychotherapists, etc.), at all career levels, to better understand this complicated area of medicine and thus be able to promote best suited treatment practices to repair the anticipated anatomic and chemical brain changes responsible for this serious problem. Furthermore, this monograph will hopefully further stimulate and enhance student and in-training health professional interest to attract others to this less often considered but extremely important area of healthcare specialization.

In this way, I feel that this monograph can and will promote further quality information usage, exchange, and discussion among providers in this field of medicine and ultimately support additional discovery, continual improvement of best medical practices, advanced interventions, and treatment standardization to allow long-term sobriety while decreasing relapse and overdose tendencies.

Acknowledgments

Finally, a heartfelt thank you to Dr. Eduardo Borges, a neurologist, whose helpful thoughts and comments throughout the entire writing process were so much appreciated. Also to Joslyn Paguio and Rebeka Henry at Elsevier publishers, who so carefully and professionally edited this book.

Overview of Book

A practical and easy to read manual for addiction treatment providers at all educational and career levels to better understand the complicated fundamentals of substance abuse and addiction. Incorporated are current applicable concepts of brain function, both normal and changes that occur from substance abuse, early management and long-term treatment protocols evolved through the unique training and extensive experience of the author, with the purpose of complimenting the more academic, lengthy, and formal publications currently available through the American Association of Addiction Medicine and other publications.

This manual emphasizes a practical and simplified understanding of the associated brain chemistry alterations, successful outpatient pharmacologic detoxification treatments, useful and effective psychiatric comorbidity drug therapy, learned and applied in consultation with the author's psychiatric and mental health counseling colleagues, a teaching review of common substance abuse associated infectious diseases and counseling strategies for affected individuals, smoking cessation protocols using substitution therapy, e-cigarettes and medication, point of care and laboratory urine substance and validity testing and interpretation, plus long-term outpatient medication management options for people using one or more commonly abused substances.

Robert D. Lovinger, MD

Contents: Overview

SECTION 1
Introduction
A summary of the fundamentals of the growing substance abuse/addiction epidemic and an introduction to understanding the associated anatomic changes, continuous alterations in brain chemistry, and the physiologic consequences from unremitting substance-induced brain damage. Discussion within this section focuses on how substance abuse destabilizes normal brain tissue; abuse and addiction time frames; neurotransmitters; early-in-life aversion strategies; nerve conduction and its resultant aberrant neurotransmitter patterns; pain categories and pain management; fundamentals of pharmacotherapy, diversion control, and other helpful corrective substance abuse modalities; and the problematic roles played by addicted patients, insurers, drug manufacturers, and physicians in addressing this overwhelming public health crisis.

SECTION 2
A Brief Guide to High-Complexity Testing for the Detection of Common Substances of Abuse in the Urine and Useful Clinical Interpretation of These Procedures
A brief guide to high-complexity abused substance-based toxicologic urine testing. Included is relevant immunoassay and mass spectrometry methodology for common substances of abuse and validity testing to detect adulteration or possible tampering with the urine sample obtained. Useful clinical interpretation of each of these procedures based on expected metabolite and time frame changes for each detected substance and validity "promote best practice clinical decision formation."

SECTION 3
Addiction Management Protocols
Author developed and tested addiction management protocols for opiates including both complete detoxification and medication-assisted treatment (MAT) are incorporated, in addition to those for alcohol, cocaine amphetamines, and other "uppers"; benzodiazepines and other sedative/hypnotics; marijuana and synthetic marijuana substances; anabolic steroids and inhalants; hallucinogens; and dissociatives.

Helpful treatment medications for comorbidities, originally suggested and successfully applied by the author's psychiatric and mental health colleagues are also included plus practical thoughts and suggestions from the author's experience concerning certain special populations that he has had the privilege of managing.

SECTION 4
Addiction Management Protocols: Smoking Cessation Management
Included are a review of commonly encountered problems faced by nicotine users, use of substitution therapy, e-cigarettes, and prescription medication treatment. Helpful suggestions are made for optimal use of each therapeutic classification discussed.

SECTION 5
Addiction Management Protocols: Long-Term Medication Abstinence Options to Help Curb Substance Abuse Relapse
This section contains optimized relapse treatment use applications, costs, and advice for each recommended drug or combinations thereof. All are discussed with an emphasis on author experience combined with recommendations from the current medical literature.

SECTION 6
Common Substance Abuse—Associated Sexually Transmitted Diseases
An up-to-date review of sexually transmitted diseases is commonly associated with substance abuse behaviors. Emphasis is placed on helping healthcare professionals to better understand these diseases, both their etiology and transmission, and thus enabling them to translate this knowledge into practical patient advice, teaching, counseling, and treatment options.

Contents

Introduction

Addiction resulting from illegal or controlled substance abuse is an overwhelming and crippling chronic brain disorder. Because of repetitive reinforcement by the continued misuse of psychoactive substances, normal brain function slowly deteriorates. This results in the onset and increasing series of new, compulsive, overpowering, personally disastrous behaviors by the affected individual.

These adaptations from the chemically induced changes in brain chemistry and anatomy (both through impairment and disorganization from noxious substances) cause previously established healthy impulse control to diminish and self-destructive actions to dramatically increase.

These powerful, new, self-destructive types of stimuli, emanating from the substance-altered central nervous system (CNS), slowly become able to produce intense, unremitting cravings which the person is unable to stop despite all efforts to do so. These cravings now produce only the uncontrollable demand for an uninterrupted fresh infusion of the necessary chemical substance(s) being clamored for by the addicted individual. The ability to organize and structure both logical and pragmatic thought processes which could previously be made by certain key, but now disordered higher function areas of this organ, has presently been lost.

The continuous need for relief from these intense cravings, once addicted, will remain until they are again temporarily satisfied by the replacement substance(s), needed by the abuser ("a fix") to stop the overstimulation of these specifically affected brain receptors. This now becomes the only way to forestall or prevent the terrifying, well-known, adverse, and debilitating effects of chemical withdrawal ("dopesick") behavior, which will be expected in an addict if the essential, required substance(s) cannot be obtained in time.

The continuous need to locate and consume these substances, rather than facing the always looming and incapacitating negative consequences of failure to do so, quickly becomes more and more predominant in an addicted individual's daily activities, as it proceeds to increasingly take over and ultimately control his/her entire life.

Thus, once addicted, an individual's life is truly in total disarray, without meaning or direction, leaving them with feelings of hopelessness and helplessness, habitually in poor health with medical and dental issues due to inattention and economic problems. This is often compounded by housing, judicial, and employment bias, increasingly prone to abuse, in addition to one or more, often severe, psychiatric comorbidities, which commonly occur due to their substance abuse–initiated brain alterations.

This unhealthy, destructive process is habitually reinforced by each act of misjudgment by the now seriously debilitated brain in order to attain the necessary, short-term, minimal beneficial or pleasurable cerebral rewards and stop the previously mentioned, overwhelming cravings and otherwise inescapable, terrifying withdrawal behaviors.

In addition to the patient, one must not forget the often devastating nightmare that addiction also presents to the rest of the immediate family. The initial family reaction, out of love and caring, is usually to try to help the addicted individual. However, this often leads to enabling or codependent types of behaviors which can seriously affect or even destroy the proximate family emotionally and financially until they come to the painful realization that they can only be supportive when the patient is attempting to "do the right thing" and must be nonsupportive when the patient does not.

DEFINITION OF ADDICTION

Addiction is not only related to illegal substance abuse but also appears in other forms.

Addiction is defined in the dictionary as a quality or condition of being addicted. Thus, it is important to think of this process as not only being applied to illegal substances but also to many other substances or activities that will dramatically stimulate the pleasure-enhancing areas of the brain and compulsively bring on feelings of exhilaration. Although these are not discussed in this book, it can occur from commonly available and legal substances such as sugar, often considered the most addictive of all chemicals, chocolate, and even excessive eating. Activity-based addictions such as gambling, sex, electronics, and shopping/hoarding are also thought to emanate from these brain areas.

Interestingly, despite the clearly detailed description of this medical problem above, addiction is not classified as a current DSM-5 diagnosis. DSM-5 diagnoses only contain criteria for a substance abuse disorder (SUD) or opiate use disorder depending on the substances used. Hopefully, in the author's opinion, this possible oversight will be remedied with a more comprehensive criteria selection for this chronic brain derangement in DSM-6 (for clarification of the distinction between substance dependence [either psychological or physiological], where a patient needs and uses long-term potentially addicting substances for a medical condition but does not develop the addictive brain changes and thus is still capable of good judgment or decision-making and can function normally in their home and work environment, and true addiction, where their overwhelming compulsion for one or more of these substances caused by brain damage from its use makes it impossible for them to successfully function in society, see comments of FDA commissioner Scott Gottlieb in the Medication-Assisted Treatment [MAT] portion of section 3).

ANATOMIC BRAIN CHANGES

An explanation of how these damaging alterations may occur in specific brain areas is due to the fact that, anatomically, the brain may be thought of as consisting of two different but inseparable and integrated components or regions/parts, each primarily controlling different CNS functions.

The first component is the white matter that includes the inner areas of the brain and spinal cord. This component is considered to be the more primitive brain area as it can be found in early evolving species. Functionally it is considered to be a communications pathway, sending electrical and chemical signals up and down the spinal cord between the body and the brain.

The second component is the newer emerging gray matter, which actually covers the inner white matter. It is generally found on the front and sides of the outside of the brain (forebrain). It contains the higher, complex functioning brain systems, which include the cerebrum, embracing such areas as the frontal cortex, which predominantly appears in later evolving animal species, in addition to the other component of the forebrain known as the diencephalon. The most notable parts of this brain area, concerning addiction, are the amygdala, hypothalamus, and the limbic system. These latter areas essentially sit between the white and gray matter, with extensive connections in both directions, and are thought to play a major role in emotional expression, some types of memory, reward, avoidance, and learning behaviors (Fig. 1.1).

Contained within the more primordial white matter are the well-developed survival-type behaviors, concerned only with critical life-preserving activities such as eating, drinking, pain control, and procreation. The newer, gray matter—developed systems possess the continually evolving higher and more complex function processes, which clearly distinguish humans from other less sophisticated, though intelligent, animal forms (e.g., higher-level decision-making,

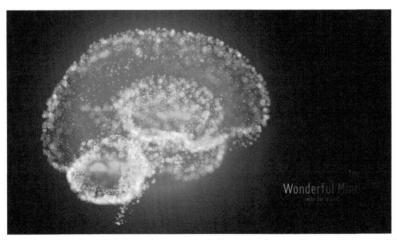

FIG. 1.1 Illustration of location of white and gray matter in the brain. Gray matter is on top and white matter in the center and then descends into the spinal cord.

judgment, impulse control, motivation, memory, augmented reward sensations, creativity and learning, advanced problem-solving, and feelings of extreme pleasure).

CHEMICAL ALTERATIONS

Medical research has revealed that within these later evolving systems, there appears to be a large number of receptors (proteins to which substances can bind or attach), which then have a capability to foster the manufacture and release of a number of chemicals called neurotransmitters that can communicate with other brain cells, two of which are dopamine, called the "pleasure or reward" chemical, and serotonin, which is also involved in this reward reinforcing process. It is most interesting that dopamine release can also be mildly stimulated or activated by a naturally pleasurable experience encountered by an individual (e.g., listening to music, exercise, chocolate, sexual activity) with later experienced long-term gratification contentment or learning from the experience.

However, addictive drugs such as opioids, cocaine, or alcohol are capable of releasing very large amounts of dopamine, which will produce extreme pleasure, but for some as yet unknown reason, does not produce long-term learning but only a maladaptive need to persistently reinforce the short-term substance-induced effect.

These chemicals, especially dopamine, are also important in the initiation, organization, and execution of the higher function processes, including motivation, learning, cognitive control, and pleasure/reward stimulation that are within and controlled by the frontal gray area of the brain. Some other key receptor-stimulating neurotransmitter (neuromodulator) systems of the at least 100 currently known and affected by both natural brain hormones and abused substances include GABA, glutamate, acetylcholine, norepinephrine, and epinephrine.

As a group, once produced by a stimulated receptor, these chemicals have been found to be capable of transmitting stimuli (excitatory or inhibitory chemical and electrical impulses) throughout this organ, which are necessary for all types of brain functioning. (When considering substances of abuse, their addicting and harm potential is based/ranked on the amount of receptor-activated dopamine that each is able to produce.) The most addicting and harmful is considered to be heroin, which is capable of increasing the amount of dopamine in the brain's reward system by 200%. This is then followed by cocaine, nicotine, barbiturates, and alcohol.

TRANSITION TO DEPENDENCE AND ADDICTION

Regrettably, the transition to dependence and then possible true addiction can start within one or only a few days of substance use. In addition, owing to continuation of recreational consumption, the diversion/misuse, and longer than necessary use of prescription medications, the incidence of this transition will increase. These debilitating brain alterations have been shown to occur in all age groups. Included are not only previously mentioned recreational consumption and diverted prescription medications but also long-term use of opiates or other controlled medications, which have been initially directed toward the alleviation of pain from trauma, chronic disease, surgery, emotional stress, or other (e.g., psychiatric) medical problems as reported by the Centers for Disease Control (CDC) and others. Thus, in the author's opinion, it is important that all potentially abusable medications must be kept under strict supervision (or equivalent) and certainly kept away from children or animals by the intended user to prevent misappropriation or accidental ingestion. The above is strongly supported by the following published facts, which sadly note the following: (1) 21%−29% of patients prescribed opiates for chronic pain misuse them or keep them in a place where diversion can easily occur, most often methadone, oxycodone, and hydrocodone; (2) more than 2 million people in the United States suffer from prescription-related abuse disorders involving opiates, and more than 100 of those are treated daily in emergency departments; (3) 4%−6% of abused prescription opioid users eventually transition to heroin or more recently loperamide (Imodium), a peripheral opioid μ-receptor agonist, often because of cheaper cost and availability; (4) fatal opioid overdose deaths from extremely powerful synthetic opioids have now passed prescription opioid deaths in number; (5) even children prescribed opioids for injuries, etc., are not immune from this problem; and (6) half the opiate prescriptions come from primary care providers.

Addictive substances, once introduced into the body, will first pass into the bloodstream and continue through the blood−brain barrier. Once inside the brain (and/or cells within the organs of the body with receptors to that particular substance), they can become attached/bind to these receptors (as previously noted, proteins on the surface of the cells that are able to grab on to that particular substance) to activate that receptor which produce the production and secrete one or more neurotransmitters, whose effect(s) then result in changes in cellular function. Concerning opiate pain control function and addiction, this involves the μ, κ, and δ receptors (with μ being the most important stimulator of the neurotransmitter dopamine), which are naturally and expansively distributed throughout the CNS and the organs within the rest of the body.

In the case where dopamine or another neurotransmitter is stimulated by an addictive substance, these chemicals can cause excessive stimulation of a certain critical brain area. In the case of opiate-related receptor activation, increased dopamine release can inordinately stimulate the appropriate neuronal systems to initiate both the desired pain palliation and/or euphoric effect (Fig. 1.2).

Besides brain receptor stimulation by environmental or laboratory-produced chemicals (e.g., addiction substances), the brain has the capacity to produce its own hormones, which can also bind to the same receptors as abused substances and function similarly by neurotransmitter stimulation and release. However, these chemicals are less potent in their functional effect due to the ability to only produce a smaller amount of a particular neurotransmitter. These chemicals are exemplified by the endorphins, enkephalins, and dynorphins. This is the system that functions in nonaddicted individuals.

In the United States, the types and numbers of substance use disorders are subject to marked geographic variation. In addition, no age groups have been spared from this increasing epidemic.

PREVALENCE AND TRENDS

Alcohol abuse is said to have a prevalence of about 8%. Furthermore, a substantial increase in alcohol consumption during the last decade has been detected, especially in women, minorities, older adults, and those socially disadvantaged. The result of increased alcohol consumption in these populations has culminated in an increasing death rate from liver disease, especially in younger people, 25—34 years of age.

Opiate addiction can be found in 2%—3% of the US population (about 2 million people) and continues to rapidly accelerate in both teens and adults. In addition, the CDC estimates that at least 50 million people or 20% of US adults suffer from chronic pain. Because of either prescribed or diverted opioid analgesics for this condition, once addicted, many then turn to either the more potent heroin or synthetic opioids (especially fentanyl analogues) for continued "relief" from this new problem that they now must face. In addition, owing

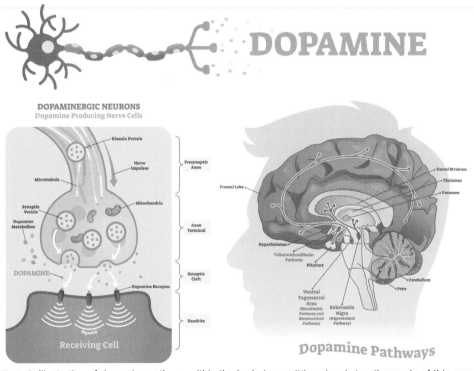

FIG. 1.2 Illustration of dopamine pathway within the brain transmitting signals to other parts of this organ. Other neurotransmitters work in a similar fashion.

to desperation, opiates originally prescribed for pets are illegally being diverted to human use. Furthermore, about 22 million people needed treatment for addiction in 2016, but only 10% of those received it, and in 2017 the CDC reports that there were 72,000 deaths from substances—about a 10% increase from the last year. Finally, substance abuse and substance overdose currently account for a skyrocketing proportion of treatment time in the emergency department, one-third of inpatient hospital costs, and about 20% of overall deaths.

It has been clearly demonstrated that all opiate compounds capable of fully stimulating opiate brain receptors are equally rewarding and potentially addictive as other non—substance-induced desirable reward behaviors (e.g., eating, drinking), which use similar brain circuits to release certain neurotransmitters, especially dopamine. This also appears to be true for other substances. However, substance potency, method of absorption, and rapidity of brain dispersion (into the reward circuit areas), in addition to the aggregate amount of usage, are also thought to be important/contribute to the rapidity of addiction conversion.

Smoking, injecting, snorting, rather than ingesting these substances will result in a speedy and more rapid rise and fall in the brain levels and dispersion of that particular drug (and also produce associated brain changes). This may also result in a more quickly addicted individual.

Furthermore, the low street price of the more potent opiate heroin and the introduction of the inexpensive, covertly produced, extremely potent, synthetic opiate compounds, mostly from the Far East through Mexico, which can be consumed either in their native form or infused into heroin or other opiate formulations to make them more potent and intense are still cheaper than most opiate-containing pills. This is the reason why these drugs are so much more "popular and deadly" among younger addicts as opposed to other available but more expensive and tougher to easily obtain prescribed opiate preparations.

The incidence of opioid-related overdoses has become a major public health crisis as the death toll rises rapidly with about 90—110 people dying each day. Furthermore, death from this substance is now higher than any other cause in people under 50 years of age. In fact, in 2015, opioid drug overdoses accounted for more than 33,000 deaths, about half from prescription, and this number continues to grow rapidly (overdoses have quintupled since 1999), creating a drop in US life expectancy. Furthermore, the CDC reports that in 2017, more than half of opioid

deaths were caused by newer extremely powerful clandestine laboratory—manufactured synthetic opioids. Finally, opiate use has now a higher death toll rate than that of automobile accidents, gun violence, or military fatalities in both Vietnam and current conflicts. Future estimates have been tragically projected to kill up to 0.5 million or more people in the next decade, especially those without appropriate access to effective and proven successful intervention modalities.

Finally, there is an increasing occurrence of comorbid opiate, benzodiazepine, and/or alcohol abuse and mortality. Opiate and alcohol comorbid deaths often start with binge drinking, which, as with benzodiazepines, due to their CNS depressant propensities, is more potentially lethal than either alone.

Cocaine, another highly abused substance, is now reported to be second in line as far as addiction goes, when compared with opioids. This is due, as previously noted, to its dopamine-stimulating abilities.

THE CONSEQUENCES OF SUBSTANCE ABUSE

The consequences of substance abuse and addiction are quite well known and include distressing health impairment (including organ disease and cancer), severe financial stress, social/psychological/psychiatric problems, injury, serious accidents, multiple overdoses and relapses, disordered brain chemistry, criminal behavior, "doctor shopping," social isolation, and an increased risk of suicide, especially in this population (addiction) and those with chronic pain and mood disorders.

The incidence and severity of these problems continues to escalate rapidly during the addiction process as brain chemistry becomes more and more distorted and inhibitory control deteriorates. In addition, there is mounting evidence that the timing and amount of brain change disparities may exist between men, women, racial, and various ethnic groups.

Recently, abuse-deterrent drug formulations (ADFs), of especially commonly prescribed opiates, have come on the market to attempt to facilitate a decrease in abuse rates. The methods used are the creation of "barriers" within the opiate formulation so that they cannot be crushed, placed into solution, or chewed. However, although safer, these formulations have thus far not been proven to be a real abuse deterrent as they have not been considered cost-effective, which would be helpful and necessary to better promote their use.

Addiction, as previously defined, is now considered a chronic degenerative CNS disease/brain disorder and not just a social aberration/criminal choice, as it is usually long-lasting, frequently lifelong, and often accompanied by multiple relapses, despite episodes of seeming detoxification and recovery. It must further be noted that similar to other chronic illnesses (e.g., diabetes, asthma), successful treatment, control, or cure is always the goal but is often difficult or impossible to obtain. Therefore, proper evidence-based sobriety treatment demands a multifaceted, shared decision-making approach, which includes similar chronic care—based, long-term insurance coverage, currently afforded to all other chronic illnesses.

INTRODUCTION TO THE PROCESS OF DETOXIFICATION AND REHABILITATION TREATMENT

Current comprehensive treatment or drug detoxification is a three-step process as described by the US department of Health and Human Services, including evaluation, stabilization, and helping place dependent patients into an appropriate level in their treatment program.

During the evaluation process, it is extremely important to state that addicted individuals are notoriously "loose with the truth." This involves disinformation and denial by the patient, which must be taken into context by the treatment team. In addition, there are many occasions where the patient is on clandestinely infused substances which he/she knows nothing about. These also may influence the treatment management step process placement level.

In addition, treatment has currently been directed toward a revival in the alternative use of MAT, using one of three medications proven to stop opioid cravings long term, a small amount of the drug buprenorphine (a partial, not a full opiate receptor stimulant), methadone (a weaker full-opioid agonist), or naltrexone (an opioid antagonist) after opioid detoxification, rather than the usual or traditional complete abstinence program not coupled with the use of long-term anticraving medications. These medications are all used in conjunction with simultaneous behavioral therapy and brain stimulation techniques for opiate addiction treatment. MAT is now becoming increasingly popular and now considered "the gold standard" as it has been shown to decrease opioid mortality and morbidity (e.g., cravings, withdrawal, overdose, and relapse by more than half) when compared with complete abstinence programs without follow-up anticraving medication use. The use of one of these medications, after detoxification from other opioids, will now enable this previously opioid-addicted person, currently craving free, to again function normally in society and the workplace on a daily basis (see comprehensive discussion of MAT in section 3), but it must be recognized that unfortunately, current harm reduction strategies do not work for everyone and thus not prevent all substance abuse deaths. Finally, it must also be noted that MAT medications do not work for everyone with opiate addictions, and other long-term alternative medication treatments are also currently available (see section 5).

In the author's opinion, it is extremely important that all-inclusive initial efforts should focus on early-in-life primary prevention to thwart, curb, or successfully treat substance experimentation or diversion in late childhood or early adolescence to discourage our youth from potentially starting on the road to dependence or addiction, and possible lifelong brain injury. Unfortunately, present efforts in this regard have, thus far, been inadequate and therefore predominantly unsuccessful.

As indicated above, new achievement-oriented programs are in desperate need of development. In fact, it has been reported that only one in four adolescents and young adults received an evidence-based medication for their addiction, and the gap was much larger in the adolescent population alone. Furthermore, those who received one of these medications were much more likely to remain engaged in treatment which included a combination of innovative late childhood behavioral health or early adolescent initiated self-help strategies, including aversion, diversion control, dissemination of substance reduction information or public and provider education, plus community- and family-based interventions such as mental health services, various modes of mental health therapy, and other similar resources.

In addition, the use, incorporation, or expeditious adoption of efficacious chemical supplements, chemotherapeutic medications (pharmacotherapy), smoking cessation treatment, aerobic exercise/yoga/palates, acupuncture, spiritual, and short- and long-term linked cognitive/behavior modification/psychological/psychiatric, and 12-step rehabilitation measures has been found to be enormously helpful at all stages of prevention or treatment.

Other potentially helpful measures currently being researched include vaccines able to produce antibodies to abused substances with the hope of preventing attachment of these chemicals to their brain receptors. Thus, stimulation of these proteins cannot occur. In addition, research in reference to immune system produced proteins, to combat addiction by altering the desire to use substances (e.g., granulocyte colony-stimulating factor, G-CSF), is also in development as are brain mapping technologies to document both initial concerns and treatment success.

Finally, repetitive transcranial magnetic stimulation (rTMS) for treating SUDs using electromagnets on the head and thus avoiding the need for a chemical to pass through the blood-brain barrier is being developed and appears encouraging. Their mechanism of action has recently been better elucidated and is acknowledged to help correct the substance-induced abnormal neuroadaptive brain connections and frontal reward system changes. In this regard, the FDA has recently approved a nerve stimulator, NSS-2 Bridge, worn behind the ear for about 1 week to help mitigate withdrawal, pain, anxiety, depression, and sleep problems for those dealing with opiate (and possibly other substance-induced) debilitating, withdrawal symptoms.

Also considered essential are family, school, social, and community reconciliation strategies. These have now replaced the simpler, traditionally available, abrupt, somewhat forceful, antiquated, inadequate, impassionate, therapeutically unproven, slipshod, "cold turkey" type sobriety efforts, alone. This detoxification modality is still being employed in some programs but obviously less successful in deterring or thwarting relapse and possible overdose in affected patients.

Organizations such as Alcoholics Anonymous and Narcotics Anonymous are also beneficial to recovering addicts to facilitate and help them better navigate the road to reestablishing lost connections with old friends and family, making new friends, helping to overcome possible substance-induced long-term personality changes, in addition to reassociating and regaining the ability to contribute to society in a wholesome and healthy manner. However, these already available education or intervention-based strategies are still in need of further innovative development and consensus-based standardization.

As previously indicated, the reason thought to be responsible for the initiation and continuation of these chronic behaviors involves the ability of the brain to gradually, but somehow adversely transform or change itself through altered structural and neural activity. These increasingly abnormal adaptations of the brain's extremely complex interconnections (neuroadaptations) induce the generation of new, but faulty, homeostatic changes within the original brain circuitry to reset the system within the principal regions of decision-making, impulse, pain, motivation and reward, behavioral control contained in the limbic

and infralimbic cortex system (for cocaine), or its extensions and prefrontal and frontal areas of this organ.

As previously stated, the once normal brain becomes increasingly dysfunctional as chemical abuse continues, leading to an escalating risk of dependence and addiction. This is especially important in adolescents, young adults, military personnel, and veterans, as early substance abuse can interfere with normal CNS development. In fact, the greatest risk for lifelong substance dependence or addiction occurs in those aged 14 years and younger who begin their substance use/abuse at that time, often first using one or more of the "so-called" gateway drugs (marijuana, alcohol, and nicotine), which are associated with feelings of substance reinforcement and reward, which they then want to maintain. In this population, the brain may also be unable to properly complete its normal development or maturation, which characteristically persists until the age range of 20–25 years. In fact, the author believes that is why many of his patients in their mid-late 20s act like young teenagers.

The good news is that while experimentation with substances is common at younger ages, most who try them will stop their use and do not go on to eventually reach a problematic use and/or CNS impairment stage.

PATTERN OF ADDICTION PROGRESSION

After speaking with a large number of patients throughout the author's numerous practice years, there appears to be a commonly cited pattern of three overlapping phases in the acute addiction development cycle.

Initially, these patients characteristically begin the addiction process with physician-prescribed or diverted substance use to try to alleviate severe physical or emotional pain or are often prompted to try a particular drug or chemical by a friend or acquaintance on a recreational basis. Once started, this individual may, over time, develop a strong need to experience and reexperience the analgesic, pleasure/wanting, reward, or euphoric response to this particular substance. This is generally referred to as drug dependence as they are still able to function successfully at home and in society.

Substance abuse then continues into the second phase, due to either the return of the original hyperalgesia (pain) or the effect of increasing tolerance, which may be defined as decreasing brain sensitivity to one or more substances being used. Thus, increasing amounts or enhanced potency/strength of the ill-used drug(s) must now be consumed to try and reproduce the pretolerance developed "high" or pain relief. This is a common practice during the "cutting or adulteration" process by the drug dealers who wish to both increase their profits and retain each "client" during this later tolerance phase by the supplementation or addition of stronger or other psychoactive substances (one of these is levamisole, an antiparasitic medication which is partly metabolized to an amphetamine-like compound capable of increasing dopamine concentration in the reward pathway). Others are very strong manufactured opiates (e.g., fentanyl derivatives).

Within this phase, the possibility of an overdose and the likelihood of potential mortality increases as a result of the well-described, drug-induced breathing cessation (especially with the new, extremely potent opiate analogue substances currently available where only a grain of the substance can result in overdose and death, as discussed later in this section). However, despite the increased amount or potency of the substance(s) used, the initial pain or elation response begins to start decreasing incrementally, and cravings become predominant, leading to the beginning of the state of true addiction, which may be best characterized by more than just physiological dependence but by the need to compulsively use the substance despite the increasing lack of concern for self-harm.

They then enter the third phase where they are usually unable to fully experience the original euphoric feelings or pain relief but must now face the inability to stop the use of these substances because of the overwhelming fear of the impending, intense, severe, and inevitable withdrawal symptoms which will appear sometime in the near future (few hours). The consequence of this phase is to increase drug-seeking behavior at any personal cost.

These phases may also be conceptually interpreted from a chemical standpoint.

NEUROTRANSMISSION: CHEMICAL AND ELECTRICAL STIMULATION

Although this is a very complicated and still not a fully understood process, stimulation of most brain and/or spinal cord receptor proteins is usually thought to be controlled by the previously discussed abused substances (e.g., opiates) or endogenous chemical messengers (e.g., endorphins). They then stimulate these specific receptors to release neurotransmitters. The chemicals (neurotransmitters) liberated by the stimulated receptors are then able to initiate and send electrical signals to other nerve cells that they come in contact with until they reach their final destination.

It is most interesting, as previously pointed out, that substances of abuse appear to be able to exert their clinical inhibitory or excitatory effects through the stimulation of appropriate receptors, which then is capable of markedly increasing the secretion of one of the many endogenous neurotransmitters made within the cell and stored in small sacs (called synaptic vesicles) in the membrane at the end of the nerve cell.

Once expelled by stimulation into the space between contiguous nerve cells (called the synaptic cleft), the neurotransmitter then opens small channels at the top of the next cell in the chain. The amount of neurotransmitter discharged onto the cleft will determine how long the channels in the next cell will be open and thus denoting the amount of time the neurotransmitter is able to stimulate the receptor of the next cell (and influence the signal strength). The neurotransmitters are then either destroyed by certain chemicals (enzymes) which are active in the synaptic cleft or again taken back up into the cell that originally discharged it and restored in the original sac until again stimulated to send another nerve signal. This mechanism allows the chemical messages to then stimulate the creation of electrical impulses which pass through the cell and stimulate the next cell in the nerve pathway to reach its ultimate destination (s) within the brain and/or body.

Once there is a basic understanding of nerve transmission and the important role of neurotransmitters in this process, attention can now be turned to how aberrations or derangement in the normal nerve transmission process may be related to the development of substance abuse patterns.

It now becomes easy to realize that if one of the effects of addictive substances is to block the reuptake transport of both dopamine and serotonin (which they do), and therefore prolong their time of stimulation (preventing the turnoff of the dopamine signal) or reinforcement on the next nerve cell in the pathway, the deleterious consequences caused by these abnormal chemical processes can make sense in its role as one of the keys in both the development and continuation of addiction from excessive stimulation of the brain's reward circuit.

Another important recent discovery concerning the ability to produce addictive behaviors is the role played by the immune system within the brain. This system is controlled by the glial cells within this organ, which act to keep our brains healthy. However, it has now been established that many substances are capable of binding to receptors within these cells and then transforming/causing the ability to subvert normal protective action to foreign substances by generating increasing abnormal immune-like signals, which then amplify the reward-generating properties of dopamine. One of these immune receptors that has already undergone significant study is toll-like receptor 4 (TLR4).

As indicated above, neurotransmitters can be either inhibitory or excitatory by altering the strength of the electrical signal from one cell to another. Furthermore, a cell is capable of producing either one or more than one neurotransmitter(s), which it can then send into the synapse to influence the strength of the electrical signal going to the next cell or cells in the chain (Figs. 1.3 and 1.4).

In the case of opiates, the original substance introduced into the body can either attach directly to an opiate receptor (μ, κ, or δ—with μ being the most formidable in producing its pleasurable clinical effects) or use an intermediary natural hormone such as an endorphin, to accomplish its clinical impact in the brain. Dopamine can also produce or increase other psychostimulant (e.g., cocaine, amphetamine) effects in that organ.

It is also important to understand, as previously implied, that opiates and other substances of abuse are also able to send signals via multiple distinct pathways to the pleasure or reward areas within the frontal lobes, the specific recognized receptors within the body organs, and the respiratory area in the posterior part of the brain, or both targets, therefore initiating the usual CNS functions (both positive and deleterious), which may originate in these areas within the brain.

Synaptic transmission

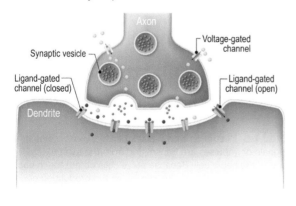

● Na⁺   ● Neurotransmitter   ○ Ca²⁺

FIG. 1.3 Detailed illustration of a synapse showing mechanism of chemical activity including production, release, and transfer/attachment to target cell receptor.

BRAIN OXYGEN STARVATION

As a consequence of the stimulation of these signal pathways, opiates (and other abused substances) can trigger/be responsible for the occurrence of an "overdose" which involves inhibition/blockage/suppression of the automatic breathing center in the back of the brain near the spinal cord called the brain stem (medulla and pons). Signs and symptoms of breathing difficulty include labored breathing (choking, gasping, or wheezing), gurgling, vomiting, inability to speak, clutching throat, cyanosis, and passing out.

Although still not completely elucidated, it appears that there are a large number of opiate and other addictive substance receptors in the brain stem. These receptors, once stimulated, are then capable of restricting the rate or depth of breathing by signal transmission interference (e.g., similar to the manner in which they act in pain reduction), which can eventually reach the point of breathing cessation, resulting in oxygen starvation. Oxygen deprivation then may also affect other body organs and CNS function, quickly leading to permanent brain damage and/or death if not promptly corrected (within only a few minutes).

This same situation may also occur in the area of the brain where voluntary breathing is controlled. Furthermore, opiates, for example, have been found to inhibit the carbon dioxide (CO_2) sensors in the neck, which then fail to stimulate more rapid breathing as the blood CO_2 levels rise and oxygen (O_2) levels decrease, thus curtailing or not being able to send the normal body "warning signals" of the imminent danger approaching.

Finally, opiates have been found to suppress the gag reflex, which protects people from vomiting and choking while tranquilized and anesthetized from the created feelings of pleasure.

Current scientific evidence indicates that the phenomenon of tolerance also occur in the brainstem (medulla and pons) opiate receptors. It appears, however, that these particular receptors are quickly able to return to their normal state (a nontolerant state), well before other opioid receptors in the brain. This is believed to be the reason that after detoxification, reuse of opiates, using the predetoxification substance strength of the opiate, can cause the automatic breathing center receptors to be much more severely affected (become overstimulated) than the opiate receptors in other areas of the brain, resulting in overdose signs and symptoms with possible fatality. This process appears to be more common during a relapse occurring within the first 6 months after complete detoxification (especially when previously prescribed anticraving medications

Synapse

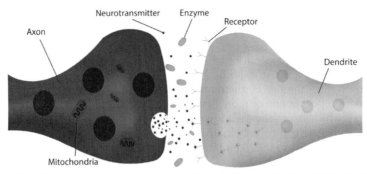

FIG. 1.4 Illustration of a synapse showing neurotransmitter release and attachment to a receptor on the next neuron in the nerve pathway.

have been voluntarily discontinued by the patient). The apparent reason for this is that the patient fails to realize that the doses used before detoxification will have a far greater effect on the breathing center than before, when he/she was in a more tolerant state.

KINDLING

Further understanding of the addiction process, as previously noted, includes the fact that serial use of these substances is also capable of increasing neuronal sensitivity (called kindling) and sustainability, though temporary, by increasing the available amount and effect of a specific neurotransmitter for a period of time.

Over time, however, these high stimulation levels from tolerance slowly start to become impossible to sustain. This is due to the brain's inability to continuously generate and secrete the same amounts of this gratification-producing or pain-controlling neurotransmitter, unless, for a while, the potency or the dose of substance taken is increased, until the brain's supply of available neurotransmitters becomes more and more depleted, but drug-seeking activity continues to remain high due to addiction.

Research has taught us that the brain is capable of producing many neurotransmitters, each one having one or more specific functions, and multiple ones can be stimulated by receptors at the same time. For example, dopamine appears to be involved with reward and pleasure, although "drug-seeking behavior" appears to be associated not with a dopaminergic process alone, but in concert with the separate glutamate neurotransmitter system (it should be noted that glutamate and acetylcholine are actually the most common neurotransmitters of the many made within this organ).

PLEASURE AND PAIN RELIEF

The pleasure or pain relief experience by opiates or natural hormones is also clearly tied to the amounts, potency, and speed of substance entry into the brain. Lipid solubility of the used substance is also an important factor in how fast brain entry occurs. (Fig. 1.5)

The natural system, which produces a lesser amount of neurotransmitter when stimulated, is the initial one activated after pain occurs, since it can function to control pain, although not to the level of a natural or synthetic opiate's capability, but again, in homeopathic amounts. Pending human trials, the use of these natural painkillers in a nasal spray formulation to quickly allow them to enter the brain is currently being evaluated for

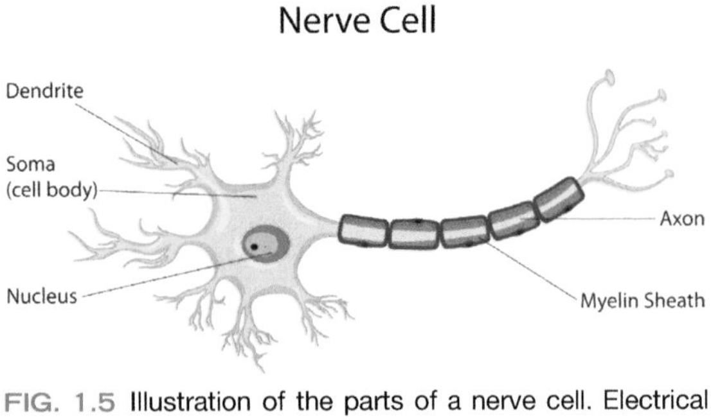

Nerve Cell

FIG. 1.5 Illustration of the parts of a nerve cell. Electrical signals or impulses are transmitted from the axon to the end of the nerve cell. Because nerve cells do not touch each other, the electrical impulse stimulates the production of chemical signals (neurotransmitters) in the nerve ending which cross the synaptic cleft or space and attach to receptors on the dendrites on the next cell in the nerve pathway. This then generates another electrical signal which will pass through this nerve cell in the chain to its end. This "domino type" of effect is then continued until the point of termination of the nerve pathway is reached.

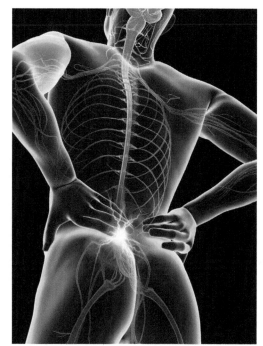

FIG. 1.6 Illustration of pain signal transmission from site of pain in body through the spinal cord to the brain.

pain management. Thus far, animal trials show that they appear to work differently than plant or synthetically produced opioids, as they have exhibited no signs of tolerance when blocking pain perception or heightened reward stimulation (Fig. 1.6).

Another chronic pain relief strategy being tried in a number of states is the use of prescribed medical marijuana to substitute, decrease, or eliminate the need for opiates. This approach uses either cannabidiol (CBD), a nonpsychoactive component of marijuana available without prescription in all states, or medical marijuana itself. Its use is currently based on the theory that it "makes sense" or is a "reasonable thing to try" to decrease the rising death rate from opiates, especially those due to the newer, extremely potent ones currently available. In addition, its use may be helpful for those with pain but who are afraid of opioids or current opiate users who want to decrease their daily dose or come off them completely, if at all possible.

Although more research into this potential alternative is essential due to the limited amount of scientific evidence already accumulated, initial studies have already indicated that neuropathic pain appears to have a positive response rate to this option. These products come in a variety of short- and long-acting formulations, including pills, creams, smokables/vapes, oils,

lozenges/sublinguals, transdermal patches, cookies, and brownies. Rapid-acting formulations such as smokables reach the brain faster, and the effects are rapid as opposed to edible formulations, which work slower but longer. Some users employ both types simultaneously for maximum length of effect.

PAIN: THE GREAT CONFOUNDER

To better understand the complex role of these abused substances, neurochemicals, and neuropeptides in the identification/assessment and treatment of pain, a few brief comments concerning pain management are in order.

1. Pain is a very complex protective process, indispensable for survival, with more than 100 types already identified in the body. It is defined by the International Association for the Study of Pain as "an unpleasant sensory and emotional experience associated with actual or potential tissue damage or described in terms of such damage." It is said that the prevalence is in the 100 million people range and to occur more frequently in people as they age.

   It is customarily recognized as being of three general types. These include cancer, which is beyond the scope of this monograph, acute, and chronic. Each type often requires a different form of treatment. (In addition, please do not forget the association between chronic pain and depression.)

2. Acute pain begins abruptly, is usually of short duration, and results from disease, inflammation, and tissue injury. Opiate therapy, because of its inherent risks, is usually not necessary, or if it is, for no more than 3 days and at the lowest possible helpful/effective doses should be used for safety reasons. Please remember that one of the important reasons to treat the pain is to prevent it from becoming longer-lasting.

3. Chronic pain is often a severe medical problem (but can be the result of an undefined cause) of longer duration and unfortunately can become resistant to many medications. In addition, it is also important to use as few CNS depressant medications at the same time for pain relief to minimize potential harmful side effects, especially respiratory depression. However, nonopioid medications (both oral and topical) or nonpharmacologic therapies (e.g., rest, tai chi for osteoarthritis, mindfulness training for osteoarthritis or chronic back pain, physical therapy, acupuncture or spinal manipulation for chronic lower back pain) are still the preferred initial

treatment modalities and should always be tried first, with opiates being used only as a second-line treatment, if necessary, when the benefits are proven to clearly outweigh the risks, and be considered, in almost all cases, for a maximum of 7 days.

4. Please remember that the long-term desire for opiate use or the start of misuse can commence within days of initiation of therapy, and the incidence of abuse increases with time.

5. Chronic pain can start as a form of acute pain and although there is no consensus on its duration before it is considered chronic. Many clinicians, however, feel it should be present for at least 6 months.

6. In general, chronic pain may be divided into two forms, the first being activation of a group of thin sensory nerves found throughout the body (especially the internal organs and skin), which respond to noxious stimuli called nocioreceptors (nocioceptive pain).

The second form of chronic pain is due to actual dysfunction or disease within the nervous system. This pain is called neuropathic pain and is not considered to be related to nocioceptive pain (Figs. 1.7—1.9).

7. Chronic pain occurs in a large portion of our population, and its intensity cannot currently be objectively measured and thus direct patient evaluation (again, the use of the CDC or state guidelines for initiation and follow-up) is extremely important. Additionally, although no accurate markers of pain are available, there are some risk assessment tools available both before and during therapy (e.g., Opioid Risk Tool, Pain Medication Questionnaire, Current Opioid Misuse Measure).

8. Nocioceptive and neuropathic pain signals can travel up and down the spinal cord and throughout

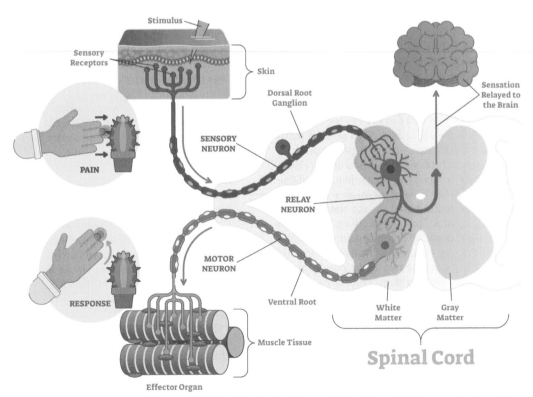

FIG. 1.7 Illustration of a reflex arc which is active in almost immediate noxious stimuli perception from the body through the spinal cord to the brain.

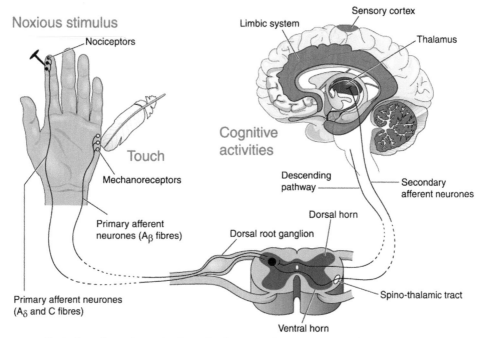

FIG. 1.8 Illustration of a noxious stimulus going from a nocioreceptor in skin through the spinal cord to the brain. The stimulus first goes to the thalamus in the central area of the brain and is then is transmitted to the cortex and/or limbic system.

the brain. The previously noted neurotransmitters within the spinal cord and brain are not only capable of signal or transmission between nerve cells but can also perform impulse modification such as blockage or enhancement of the signal/impulse. Thus, the various neurotransmitters made within the body are directly involved and responsible for pain intensity.

9. In the brain, pain signals are most often sent first to an area concerned with information storage called the thalamus, which can relay signals to other brain areas. One of these areas is the frontal cortex, which, among other things, is involved in pleasure, complex thinking, and addictions.

10. Pain management or successful treatment goals involve rebalancing neurotransmitter or neuropeptide levels, resulting in improved patient physical functioning or allowing resumption of normal participation in their usual activities of daily living.

11. A product called cannabinoid (CBD hemp oil) has recently come available. It comes from the non-psychoactive portion of the cannabis plant (little or no THC, which is found in medical marijuana). Although it is FDA approved only for the treatment of an uncommon form of childhood seizures, CBD products have been touted as a safe and natural remedy for multiple conditions such as pain, anxiety, depression, to name a few. However, in the author's opinion, the jury is still out.

12. A conceptual example of how the body might normally respond to nociceptive chronic pain signals before medication usage may be illustrated as follows:

Once pain messages from pain receptors which have become sensitized at the site of the pain within the body or in the spinal cord, they begin to fire impulses at a more rapid rate reflecting the severity of the pain. These signals, due to the process of sensitization, which can continue long after the actual pain subsides, are sent to the CNS by the appropriate neurochemical and electrical signals (e.g., substance "P") made within the body, as one or more of these previously noted neurotransmitters are produced in response to this signal. These chemicals (if there are no genetic problems which inhibit or diminish their production) then act to reduce substance "P" or other neurotransmitter release from its terminals and thus capable of diminishing the intensity of the pain signals. They are also able to block nocioceptin receptors which are involved with visceral pain.

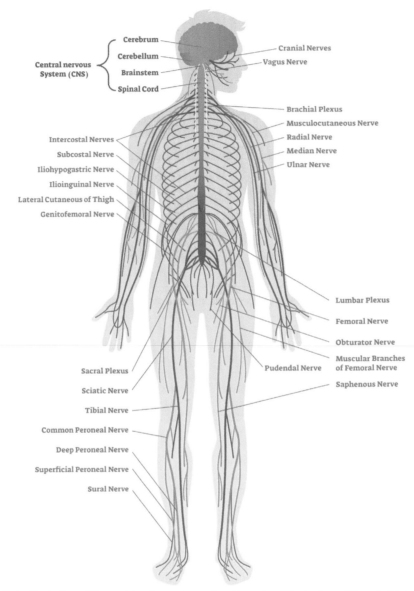

FIG. 1.9 An illustration of the peripheral nervous system throughout the body and its extensive number of pathways to the brain.

These endogenous chemicals are also capable of binding to pain receptors in the brain to block pain just as the natural and synthetic opiates do. Finally, pleasure stimulation by increasing endorphin concentrations rather than substances can also be triggered by eating certain foods (e.g., chocolate), sexual activity, aerobic exercise, and laughter.

Recent focus on new research modalities continues to provide new pain reversal solutions (therapeutic innovation, voluntary opioid tapering techniques, mechanical device(s), and/or pharmacologic discovery), which are less addictive, safer, and finally, dependence and mortality free (Fig. 1.4).

13. One recent experimental development moving in the direction of this ultimate goal is the new transdermal patch for chronic pain control, which has just been announced. It contains a high-potency CBD extract, which has all the antiinflammatory and pain-relieving effects without any psychoactive activity. Only time will tell if this will become a standard of care.

GENETIC CONSIDERATIONS

Vulnerability to substance abuse also appears to be strongly associated with the interaction of heritable genetic (40%−60%) factors, in addition to environmental agents, plus possible previous experiences that appear to also be able to modify/influence gene expression resulting in change within the brain circuitry.

These factors can, over time, begin to further influence the way this substance is perceived by the brain due to modification or changes in the receptors and genes within the brain tissue. Although still very incompletely understood, these interactive mechanisms appear to explain the way addiction propensity probably occurs. Furthermore, it explains one likely mechanism by which a potential-inherited genetic predisposition for genetic or environmentally initiated substance abuse tendencies and relapse can occur.

Early support for this mechanism has already been established due to research into the gene transcription factor, δ-FosB. It has been established that the overexpression of this heritable gene transcription factor is one of the common components in drug addiction behavior. Recent evidence in mice links 35 genes to cannabis use, certain personality types, and psychiatric conditions.

The occurrence of substance abuse and addiction is also positively correlated with the occurrence of substance-induced mental illness in affected individuals as opposed to the general population (dual diagnosis). Conversely, mental illness also increases one's susceptibility to substance abuse.

Present pharmacotherapy is focused on beneficial interventions acting at different points in the detrimental cascade of chemical interactions within the brain, to facilitate both discontinuation of the pleasurable sensations and amelioration of withdrawal symptoms caused by the substance(s) being used.

CROSS-TOLERANCE

Furthermore, it is important to remember that pharmacotherapy is based on the principal of cross-tolerance. Because of this principle, the use of one proven detoxification medication to a particular substance (e.g., using buprenorphine), a weak partial opiate agonist, can substitute for heroin or any other opiate, so detoxification or withdrawal from the abused drug(s) within this entire class of substances can be achieved (by making withdrawal less difficult/milder and/or painful).

Although addictive substances have been present on this earth longer than both the emergence of man and their discovery, use, and dependency, medical (pharmacologic) and psychotherapeutic treatment of their abuse is still in its infancy. This is due in part to the current lapse in our understanding of the previously noted genetic components of addictive behavior or the propensity thereof. In addition, past barriers to brain research are now finally becoming better elucidated with the creation of newly available technology. Additionally, our incomplete research knowledge of the possible changes in brain cell anatomy (ability of brain cells to form new connections/plasticity) and its resultant behavioral biological consequences present an additional challenge. Moreover, our slowly evolving grasp of the physiology/neuroscience of involved neurotransmitters, neuromodulators, neuropeptides, peptide hormones, receptors, and the realization that while the brain has protective mechanisms to deter potential addiction (e.g., taste, smell, discomforting feelings or experiences, pain), the recent ability to artificially produce purer, more potent substances, and the use of extremely rapid nervous system entry and precipitated drug-induced brain rise and fall concentration methodology can overcome these inborn systems, and the paucity of proven medications, which act to prevent the ultimate pleasure and addiction affects while hopefully promoting symptomless withdrawal and long-term sobriety from the used addictive substance(s) remains a significant frustration.

Although some patients (especially in the past) enter into drug rehabilitation treatment only having used a single substance, most of the patients who the author currently (as opposed to single substance abuse) treat are patients with a polysubstance abuse problem, with an often, also present mental health dual diagnosis, which has occurred either independently or most often as the result of the abused chemical (substance) itself.

BARRIERS TO RECOVERY

The clinical symptoms of each abused substance, which can occur during both the intoxicated and withdrawal state, and the accompanying either short- or long-term psychiatric/psychological comorbidities must be taken into account to better support the complex, lifelong road to recovery as substance-induced psychiatric disorders or relapses have been described long (even years) after the cessation of substance use. Common examples in the author's practice include benzodiazepines and hallucinogens.

Unfortunately, patients who undergo successful detoxification are still prone to relapse because detoxification and full recovery from substance abuse are not analogous events. In fact, after detoxification and even successful 12-step program completion, patients often continue to feel the continued effects of withdrawal for long periods of time. These effects include anxiety, depression, anhedonia (inability to feel pleasure), and even frank sadness.

The reason for this is to understand that the brain heals very slowly. By this the author means that all the anatomic changes that have occurred during the entire period of drug abuse will probably take at least as long or longer to correct. Therefore, it should be evident that the use of long-term or lifelong-duration pharmacologic relapse-prevention medication therapy, yoga, brain stimulation, exercise, etc. and psychotherapy after detoxification are extremely important to aid in recovery. However, these critical therapy components are markedly underrecommended and/or underused. In addition, the timing of the length of acute and long-term follow-up using psychological/psychiatric treatment must be matched to the individual patient as they slowly start to regain improved brain homeostasis, which may take years or an entire lifetime.

THERAPY RESISTANCE

Lastly, it is unfortunate that substance abuse patients are often reluctant or resistant to seek medical help

for this problem, thus delaying important early treatment opportunities, generally because they are not ready to resolutely confront or stop their addiction, often lie to continue obtaining prescribed opiates for their "chronic pain," or believe that substance abuse therapy is unavailable to them as it is very expensive and therefore unaffordable. In addition, much of the public still believes that addiction is an act of bad character and judgment, a moral failure rather than a medical illness, and views this population as stigmatized, dishonorable, useless, contemptible, or criminal accordingly.

Furthermore, insurance companies, government agencies, drug manufacturers, drug traffickers, and even physicians have and continue to play an illegal, enabling, and/or harmful role in this problem during the last few decades.

Insurers, because of their acute versus chronic care payment models, do not provide adequate payment for necessary detoxification and longer-term or lifelong treatment. Government agencies have failed or are financially unable to offer comprehensive funding or other acceptable healthcare options for this population. Pharmaceutical companies developed, often unethically and opportunistically, marketed the safety and efficacy of their products (e.g., the benefits outweigh the risks, especially for pain mitigation) to physicians, thus inundating the country with new and stronger (and thus more addicting) opiate formulations in addition to improperly monitoring the supply and use of prescription opiates for potentially improved financial gain. Drug traffickers continue to flood the country with heroin and other illegal cheap opioids for those who either run out of prescribed medications or believe they need stronger ones. Physicians, regrettably, have also played a significant role in this epidemic of misused opiates due to advantageous time savings by preferably writing a quick pain relief prescription, as it decreases patient contact time in the new "production line" forced reimbursement environment, increased patient contentment with the prompt nature of the pain solution, unintentional opiate overprescription, and inadequate diversion control counseling. This is supported by the CDC, National Medical Care Survey, which found that almost 30% of prescribed opioids were not supported by a pain diagnosis recorded in the prescriber's chart.

Luckily, prescribing painkilling medications has decreased markedly due to increasing amounts of available published governmental information and regulation. In addition, most doctors are inadequately trained to deal with the opioid prescribing because few medical schools teach or, at each higher level of physician training, adequately address the delicate relationship between opiate prescribing and its addiction-promoting potential. There is also failure to properly use the current (2016) CDC or state guidelines and databases for assessing and treating pain, obtaining regular urine tests on their opiate-treated pain patients, or treatment referral process gaps in their positively testing, nonopiate-prescribed patients for substance abuse treatment. In addition, only about 5% of physicians have a special license waiver to offer/prescribe buprenorphine or methadone therapy. There is also an addiction medicine educational/training handicap in understanding the correct timing and amount of substance to prescribe for a particular acute or chronic clinical problem. In addition, overprescribing of these substances often continues even though the initial benefits are clearly now outweighed by the increasing addiction risks. Finally, because of little or no training in addiction medicine by most physicians, there is little knowledge and therefore minimal confidence in the beneficial effects of the anticraving medications currently available. Thus, many physicians do not consider offering or prescribing them. In addition, they may feel uncomfortable using MAT, or anticraving medication therapy, again due to lack of training, knowledge, and experience or a less than firm understanding of this area of medicine, which includes the need for the implementation of long-term but necessary mental health or brain stimulation cotherapy.

A Brief Guide to High-Complexity Testing for the Detection of Common Substances of Abuse in the Urine and Useful Clinical Interpretation of These Procedures

INTRODUCTION

Addiction has now been proven to be a chronic brain disorder, similar to other chronic medical conditions, accompanied by numerous anatomical and chemical changes in the central nervous system, which were caused by the abused substances used. The frontal areas of the brain, containing the more recently evolving brain gray matter, where complex judgment issues are formed and executed, are one of the primary targets of these deleterious substances. The consequence of these changes results in the affected individual now being incapable, less capable, or barely able to make rational, "common sense—type" decisions concerning his/her health and welfare. Only self-preservation decisions (ex-eating, drinking, pain control, procreation) made by other brain areas, contained within the more primitive white matter, appear to be less affected at this point.

Testing Basics

Because these changes are very slow to correct, especially early in the recovery process, cravings and fears of severe, overwhelming suffering from the effects of withdrawal, in addition to continuation of substance-seeking behaviors, are still very common as the newly recovering patients enter or reenter this new sobriety phase of their lives, usually in a rehabilitation facility.

Accordingly, many admitted patients attempt to bring clandestinely hidden substances with them to "fend off" or better control these expected/anticipated problems. Abused substances are often expertly hidden in their belongings, on their bodies, or often in body cavities to avoid detection due to legal search constraints and can be used on an "as needed" or desired basis. The author has even witnessed the use of "drug-sniffing" dogs in treatment facilities to aid in hidden substance detection in addition to the usual facility-established search protocols.

Thus, serial substance abuse screening/testing is not only important for diagnosis, monitoring, minimizing falsification, relapse detection, and evaluation but also an essential, routine, and necessary measure that must be performed fairly often (although no specific number of tests have been established to date but recommended to be performed more often in the early stages of the recovery process), which must be clinically based on the needs of each individual patient, level of care, other placement considerations, and special or unique circumstances. Current test timing is usually performed to be as sure as possible that a drug-free therapeutic environment is achieved or maintained, so recovery, improved patient management, and outcomes can be accomplished or maximized. Nevertheless, these tests must only be used for medical necessity, as they are prone to overuse or lax interpretation for unlawful financial gain by unscrupulous felons.

The medical literature supports a combination of routine and "smart manner" testing using random unanticipated evaluations, based on the patient's condition, and it should be encouraged. Increased amounts of testing are recommended, as indicated above, especially early in the rehabilitation continuum (unless hampered by cost), to detect and document these substances, so clinically relevant treatment decisions, based on these findings, can be made and implemented. Urine or other tissue-type testing can also be used to encourage positive reinforcement for continued abstinence, during and after the initial recovery process, although usually at diminished levels of tests that need to be performed.

Testing for substances of dependence and abuse is important to support and monitor all short- and long-term stages/aspects of detoxification and recovery (including the time of use of long-term anticraving medications or low-dose, long-term, buprenorphine therapy [MAT]), in addition to its importance in detecting relapses during the entire process from discovery and initial treatment of substance misuse through the rest of the life of an affected individual. Thus, as with all medical tests, it is mandatory that all clinicians who deal with the substance abuse population understand its uses, benefits, and limitations.

Unfortunately, most health professionals are not well trained or versed in the sophisticated practices of substance-abusing patients nor urine toxicology interpretation, which could result in clinical decision errors (testing interpretation should only be performed by providers with expertise in urine toxicology, methodology, and clinical substance abuse management). Insurers, in the author's opinion, are also guilty of trying to dictate numbers of approved urine tests because of misunderstanding (or not attempting to understand based on reimbursement issues) the pivotal role of somewhat frequent substance abuse testing in this group of extremely brain disordered, extremely deceptive, and fragile patients, especially early on in this process.

Substance abuse testing can be accomplished by using one or more of a number of possible matrices (biological samples or specimens used for analysis), including oral fluid (sputum), blood, plasma, serum, hair, and urine. Each matrix has advantages and disadvantages including different detection time windows, sensitivity, and specificity. Nevertheless, only urine testing will be discussed, as a review of these other matrices is beyond the scope of this book.

The matrix most validated and commonly used in substance abuse treatment centers involves urine testing, using methods of high-complexity testing.

It is also important to point out that it usually takes for the kidneys at least 2 h to start eliminating an abused chemical from the body into the urine. Only then can they be detected. Therefore, testing too early can lead to erroneous or misleading results.

High-Complexity Testing
High-complexity urine testing for the presence or absence of one or more commonly abused substances and/or treatment medications, legal and illegal, is the most accurate and sensitive way of identifying, quantifying, and

tracking the expected (or nonexpected) chemical(s), during treatment management, prescribed drug administration, and the occurrence of apparent diversion or misuse. Its only limitation is its inability to pinpoint exactly when the substance was last used and the precise dose when it entered the body. It also may produce a false-negative result when the amount of a particular substance in the urine, though detectable, is below the cutoff value for that particular high-complexity test method or the substance in question cannot be successfully analyzed by the test method used. If this is the case, one cannot rule out the presence of low levels of that substance. Luckily, low levels of an abused substance are generally of little or no clinical significance.

High-complexity testing is available in two forms, each using a different chemical method of detection.

Table 1: Overview of High-Complexity Urine Testing for Substance Abuse:

Comprised of two forms, using different chemical methodology
1. Presumptive/preliminary testing
   a. Called enzyme immunoassay (EIA) testing
   b. Uses manufactured antibodies in a cup for point-of-care testing or in a laboratory where more tests are available for analysis
   c. Less accurate than confirmation testing
   d. Only gives positive or negative result
   e. Prone to adulteration
2. Confirmation/definitive urine testing
   a. "The gold standard"
   b. Uses highly complex chemical methodology
   c. Cannot be fooled or adulterated
   d. Able to determine the exact concentration of each chemical substance tested for

---

Presumptive Urine Testing
The first method of detection is called enzyme immunoassay or EIA. This method of testing uses antibodies, created in a laboratory, which are designed by the manufacturer to bind to specific biological substances (called analytes), which in this case are substances of abuse, so they can be identified. This method is very useful, especially on admission and for random testing, as it is of low cost and often informative. However, it possesses lower sensitivity and specificity (with the probable exception of the cocaine metabolite BZE) than confirmation testing, the other method of high-complexity testing. It is usually used by gathering a urine sample in a special cup containing strips (different cups may contain different number of strips) to detect each specific

substance designed for the strips to test at the designated point of care (POC): when the patient enters the program, is first awakened, being asked at any time by members of the treatment team, or when some suspicion arises (where it is especially useful). EIA testing can be performed using a cup or dipstick method, or also in a toxicology laboratory setting where the results are more accurate because of better quality control test standards. However, the results obtained by the EIA method, either at the POC or in the laboratory, are considered to be markedly less accurate than confirmation testing because they are capable of demonstrating only positive or negative (qualitative) results, which means only evidence of the presence or absence of a particular substance or one of its metabolites (breakdown products). In addition, this chemical method is vulnerable to adulteration as will be further explained later in this section. The reason for its diminished precision is that the EIA high-complexity chemistry method has still not been scientifically developed to the point where it can detect or target even a majority of the known abused substances, and it is not reliable enough to determine the total or exact amount of the expected substance (which may be present but of lower concentration than the cutoff value in the urine and thus reported as negative) from the submitted sample. Specimen-handling errors can also be the cause of incorrect results. However, it is still very helpful for initial clinical or patient management correlation. Finally, the antibodies used for each substance used in an EIA evaluation are made by a number of manufacturers. All are considered imperfect in their ability to detect each specific analyte (abused substance), as they are all somewhat different in chemical structure. Because of this, each batch of the antibodies made by every individual manufacturer is potentially capable of cross-reacting with other classes of substance with similar chemical structures. Thus, they are considered prone to producing incorrect or false/misleading results. For this reason, this method of testing is usually not considered admissible in a court of law and should only be considered as a presumptive positive requiring more definitive confirmation.

In a clinical setting, because of its potential false-positive or false-negative detection rate, it should not be overinterpreted, considered definitive, or applied in any punitive or confrontational manner unless clearly admitted by the involved patient. In addition, all products, such as herbal supplements or medications, must be reviewed and approved before the patient is allowed to continue using them because some may be capable of chemically interfering with EIA methodology.

Confirmatory/Definitive Testing

The second most currently used high-complexity method is called gas or liquid chromatography—mass spectrometry (GCMS or LCMS). Its technology is based on highly sophisticated molecular weight and charge analysis. The chromatography area of the instrument separates the specimen into all of its discrete chemicals, and the mass spectrometer then identifies each separate substance or breakdown product (metabolite) and its exact amount. LCMS instruments can also be used in tandem for better chemical separation/identification called LCMS/MS. It uses extremely complex chemical methodology for analysis. It is expensive and time-consuming, but it can definitively detect or eliminate the presence or absence (positives and negatives) of all substances of abuse for which it has been programmed, which are still within the body. In addition, prescribed medications used in substance abuse treatment are often included. Thus, it is able to exclude all false-positive tests and include all false-negative tests that it has been programmed to detect, which EIA methodology may have erroneously misidentified (this problem occurs most often in the clinical setting when presumptive positive results are disputed by a patient), plus determine their exact concentration (quantitative test) in the urine sample within the cutoff levels and window of detection time. It is usually performed after, and is generally considered to be complementary to, EIA testing (called reflex testing when it is automatically performed after presumptive testing). The GCMS or LCMS results are deemed to be definitive: "the gold standard." However, it has been prone to overuse by criminals in the substance abuse treatment industry, exploiting it only for increased financial gain.

What make this method so attractive and important when dealing with substance abuse are as follows: (1) It can detect substances the patient failed to disclose or was not capable of being detected by EIA methodology, which could affect their subsequent clinical care, and (2) it can uncover chemicals in the body that even the patient was not aware of, including those clandestinely infused into the substances that they are using, which may require further observation and/or additional treatment. In addition, precise detection of all abused substances can signify needed adjustments for any potential challenges, which may lie ahead concerning clinical decisions, medication therapy change, or change in legal considerations.

A question often asked is how often a urine test should be performed. According to recent generally accepted guidelines, the frequency and length of testing should be individualized, often using both a regular and random test schedule, and based on the level of care or patient acuity (especially during initial stabilization and tapering) rather than, as indicated before, on an arbitrary number assigned or created by an insurer, facility, or an unrelated or nonaddiction treatment management standard. In the author's opinion, arbitrary testing limits make little or no sense because each patient is constantly being assessed by multiple members of the entire treatment team. This includes physicians, nurses, multiple mental health counselors, technicians, etc. Each member of the team who feels that a reason exists to test or retest a patient should note in the patient's chart and report to the appropriate staff members who can then request an additional urine examination based on that suspicion.

Current guidelines also stress that at least a 5-year testing period, at slowly increasing time intervals, should be used to support evidence of a long-term, stable recovery.

The American Society of Addiction Medicine has recently issued their interpretation of "appropriate testing guidelines," which specifically emphasizes clinical individualization based on particular patient needs (including smart testing) rather than arbitrary payer-mandated decisions. They also take into account that the frequency of testing should be made by the ordering physician, in cooperation with the entire treatment team based on his/her judgment with the necessity of more frequent testing being performed early in the recovery process to support proof of stabilization by identifying decreasing concentrations of the substances abused by each patient after admission. Its use is also important to identify substance tampering or covert use.

Furthermore, similar increased frequency testing early on in treatment for patients with a dual diagnosis is essential to help differentiate the cause of the problem as more likely being related to the substance(s) consumed or to an underlying psychiatric illness to further help guide therapy. The additional and critical use of random (unscheduled) drug testing, so as to enhance appropriate care level placement, relapse, clinical decision-making, and reassessment, improving outcome results, in addition to maintaining the ability to render continuous high-quality patient management by the treatment team, has proven to be an additional valuable clinical tool. Finally, regional or state adjustment for specific types of substances, in the LCMS menu, commonly or frequently used in that area must also be considered, and the local appearance of new substances should be taken into account in test regimen development by each treatment facility (e.g., the use of Flacca in Florida). Moreover, the test menu should be reevaluated and adjustments made on a timely basis for each treatment facility.

Each patient admitted should have all medications and other personal products (e.g., dietary supplements) brought on admission checked for potential drug testing interactions before allowing their use.

Reasonable Testing Guidelines

In the author's experience, a reasonable general guideline is to perform presumptive (EIA) urine testing one to three times per week during the first 90 days of abstinence. After 90 days, one to three tests per month are generally adequate for clinically stable individuals but may be necessary more often in those suspected of relapse. If previously undetected substances are found, it may then require returning this patient to a higher level of care. Again, documentation is the key to this process.

What the author currently promotes, for reasons of pragmatism that are due to significant problems with certain insurer laboratory reimbursement policies, is to have a tech check the urine by the cup or dipstick method one to three times per week in a mixed scheduled and random fashion. The author uses this method because this method is inexpensive (about $3.00 per cup if commercially purchased but can often be obtained either more cheaply or even for free from the laboratory used by the treatment facility). Thus, the author generally chooses not to send out many tests to a laboratory for routine presumptive substance detection. This then eliminates any reimbursement problems with that particular insurer. Nevertheless, because of previously mentioned quality control limitations of the cup or dipstick method, accuracy is definitely compromised in comparison with laboratory-performed preliminary testing, which amplifies the need for reflex confirmation testing that the author uses about once per week for the first 90 days of sobriety or more often for cause.

If a test has one or more unexpected positive results, the author then decides, based on clinical evaluation, discussions with the treatment team, and extensive experience, whether the presumptive test needs to be sent for a confirmation test or just continue to watch the patient clinically. If sent for confirmation, the author carefully documents the need in the chart.

A full-panel, comprehensive, definitive/confirmation testing should be routinely performed, in the author's opinion, when the patient first enters and leaves a detoxification program or a lower than detoxification treatment level (PHP, IOP, or OP), as previously indicated, at least once per week routinely during the first 90 days of abstinence, to follow/compare previously detected substance levels, which in most cases should be incrementally decreasing weekly or at least every second week during the first months of abstinence. However, a routine confirmation testing done after the initial one when entering a program does not need to be as comprehensive in test numbers but more positive substance oriented as long as there is no suspicion of clandestine abuse.

Additional testing should always be performed as often as necessary for cause. It should also be used, in the author's opinion (as determined by the patient's medical insurance policy), to minimize the possibility of sending a patient to a lower level of care while still sick/unstable (especially if high levels of the previously detected substances are still present), and/or where necessary, controlled, anticraving or especially seizure control medications are no longer routinely being used.

After the first 3 months of treatment in a committed, abstinent patient, routine physician-directed confirmation tests during this period need not exceed 1–3 per month unless for cause (e.g., a new positive presumptive test) and the reason properly recorded in the medical chart.

Random (unannounced) urine testing is often the preferred testing method and should be included in each individual's regimen especially just after weekends, holidays, and passes (home visits, etc.). Random testing should always be part of the testing process to keep the patient from knowing when testing might be performed and thus discourage the possibility of clandestine substance consumption (relapse).

Please again remember that the testing frequency must meet reasonable medical necessity requirements and be documented in the physician's or clinical record if ordered by the physician or at the request of other members of the treatment team.

Table 2: Rational Urine Test Performance Guidelines:
  a. Should be individualized
  b. Use combination of regular and randomized test schedule
  c. One to three presumptive tests per week during first 90 days of sobriety
  d. Additional tests for cause or suspicion
  e. Full panel confirmatory tests on admission and discharge
  f. Abbreviated/less comprehensive, previously noted substance-oriented confirmatory test panel once per week during first 90 days of sobriety to follow abused substance levels (hopefully decreasing or dissipated)
  g. Additional confirmatory testing should be performed for cause and reason noted in patient's chart

---

Clinical Pearl

The most frequent question that the author is asked concerns the fact that all positive screening tests should be followed by a confirmation test. The answer to this question is *no* because almost all positive tests on admission will probably remain positive until the substance and/or all of its breakdown products are out of the urine. The way the author approaches positive presumptive test results is to only confirm all newly appearing positive substances in this urine test, or presumptive testing indicates that a particular substance is positive long after its presence should have disappeared. Additionally, serial weekly confirmation testing results should show only similar or lower levels of all previously positive urine tests. If the results are markedly higher on the weekly confirmation tests, then repeat confirmation testing should be considered, especially if relapse is suspected or admitted.

In conclusion, complete knowledge of the specific abused substances and their amount in urine is necessary for the treating physician and the entire therapeutic team to provide comprehensive patient-centered care, including the need and length of possible detoxification and taper, and to detect relapse or clandestine use. Furthermore, it will equip managing physicians and the rest of the healthcare team to perform best practice medicine and healthcare delivery.

In the author's effort to help healthcare team members concerning their understanding of the proper is and benefits of these urine testing methods, he has created the following concise guide, which is hoped to be both helpful and informative to assist in formulating the necessary clinical decisions to help promote a treatment protocol in the best interest of each individual patient (and hopefully avoid some of the many calls that the author currently receives from other team members concerning potentially problematic, especially EIA-completed test results). Please remember, however, that the average length of time that a substance will be found in the urine also depends in part on the length of time the substance was used pretreatment, an individual's metabolic rate, and daily amount used by the patient before treatment. Thus, the longer the amount of time of substance use and the daily amount consumed, the longer a substance may be found in the urine sample of that individual, although hopefully in diminishing concentrations over time.

OPIATES AND METABOLITES

All opiates fall into one of the three classes. These are the natural opiates, semisynthetic opiates, and the synthetic opiates.

The natural opiate group includes opium, morphine, codeine, and thebaine, which are produced by the opium poppy plant itself.

EIA methodology is very helpful, quick, and useful in detecting natural opiates, especially at the POC. However, it is unable to differentiate between any of the four natural substances. LCMS is able to fully differentiate each of the exact substances present in the urine sample and provide their total amounts.

The semisynthetic group of opiates comprises substances such as heroin, hydrocodone, hydromorphone, and oxycodone. All are made from opium poppy extracts. They need their own assays although heroin is quickly metabolized to 6-MAM and then slowly to morphine.

EIA technology is available for the detection of oxycodone, but it has not worked as well as the author would like. LCMS technology is needed to detect all others.

Synthetic "opiates" are produced in either commercial or often clandestine laboratories as they contain no opium resin. They are often much more potent than the natural varieties. This group contains the "imitation" opiates including, but not limited to, buprenorphine, butorphanol, fentanyl, levorphanol, meperidine, methadone, oxymorphone, pentazocine, and tramadol in addition to other, clandestinely produced, very potent fentanyl analogues (which may have to be tested for separately using specialized LCMS technology).

EIAs currently exist only for buprenorphine, methadone, fentanyl, meperidine, and tramadol.

As noted above, the use of urine immunoassays for high-complexity presumptive/preliminary testing is also limited because a number of common medications can produce false-positive results for opiates. These include quetiapine for methadone, naloxone for oxycodone, ofloxacin, papaverine, and rifampicin for some detectable opioids by this methodology. In addition, poppy seeds actually contain a small amount of morphine and codeine and thus can produce false-positive opiate identification.

Some opiates can only be found in the urine for a limited amount of time, further curbing the usefulness of presumptive EIA methodology. However, LCMS techniques can not only detect all opiates, even in trace amounts (if the detection limits are set very low), but also opiates are converted in the body to metabolites (breakdown products), which can be detected in the urine for much longer periods of time. The only current exceptions are the newer, extremely potent fentanyl analogues, such as carfentanil, the large animal tranquilizer, W18 and U47700, which cannot usually be identified in routine LCMS testing but can only be identified by specialized add-on LCMS configuration tests for each specific known analogue.

Finally, the normetabolites of opioid metabolism (noroxycodone, norhydrocodone, noroxymorphine, normeperidine, norfentanyl, norcodeine), which LCMS technology can identify, stay in the urine even longer. Average estimates of detection times for some opioids and metabolites are as follows. (Please again remember that the length of time that a substance will be found in the urine also depends on the previous amount of time the patient was using the opiate, the metabolic rate of the individual, and the daily amount used by the patient. Thus, the larger the time span using and the amount used daily, the longer a substance can usually be found or detected in the urine test samples of that individual.) In addition, Federal mandatory guidelines starting 10/1/17 will now require testing for oxycodone, oxymorphone, hydrocodone, and hydromorphone, which includes pain medications such as OxyCodone, Vicodin, Percocet, and Dilaudid.

General Urine Detection Time Table

Opioids and their metabolites/breakdown products in general can be detected in the urine for about 5 days.

Codeine: 1−2 days.

Methadone: used for a limited time, 2−3 days. For those on maintenance, it can be present for 7−9 days or longer.

EDDP: a methadone metabolite, can be present for up to 10 days.

Heroin: 2−4 days (be aware that heroin is rapidly converted to 6-MAM and later measured as morphine). Codeine is also partially metabolized to hydrocodone and morphine.

MAM, a specific breakdown product of heroin, is usually detected for less than 8 h. It is then converted to hydrocodone and/or morphine.

Buprenorphine can usually be found in a urine sample for 48−56 h. However, as a Buprenorphine conjugate (norbuprenorphine), 5−7 days.

Hydromorphone: 2−5 days.

Morphine: 2−4 days.

Oxycodone: 2−4 days.

Loperimide (Immodium): 8 days by LCMS

Dextromethorphine (DXM): 12 hours by LCMS

Table 3: General Detection Times of All Major Urine Substance Groups by Confirmation (GC or LCMS) Testing.

1. Opiates and metabolites:
   Generally, 5 days
   Some metabolites can be present for up to 10 days
2. Alcohol and metabolites:
   Alcohol, about 8 h
   Alcohol metabolite, up to 10 days
3. Cocaine and metabolite:
   Cocaine, about 3 days
   Cocaine metabolite, up to 15 days
4. Other stimulants: amphetamines/ Methamphetamine
   Generally 3–4 days
5. Benzodiazepines:
   a. Short acting, 1–4 days
   b. Intermediate acting, 4 days
   c. Long acting, up to several weeks
6. Marijuana and synthetic marijuana:
   a. Marijuana, 30–60 days
   b. Synthetic marijuana, 10–12 days

Alcohol, Kava, and Metabolites

Alcohol is present in the blood and urine for only a short time (about 8 h) after ingestion, unless there is delayed bladder emptying. However, one of its breakdown products, ethyl glucuronide (EtG), can be detected by using both EIA (although my experience with cross-reactivity of this metabolite has been a problem) and LCMS for days. Other breakdown products such as ethyl sulfate (in addition to EtG) can be detected by using LCMS for a few more days.

EIA assays are available to detect alcohol and EtG in the urine for generally less than 12 h. Please note that EIA testing for EtG is, in the author's experience, specifically prone to false-positive testing. This often occurs in people who use hand sanitizers and other alcohol-containing products such as mouthwash, or if the patient has elevated levels of glucose in the urine. LCMS technology is able to successfully detect alcohol metabolites (EtG, Es) in the urine for up to 5 or so days because of their slower clearance from the body.

KAVA

Kava comes from the root of a south Pacific plant. Its effects are said to be similar to alcohol, but supposedly without the hangover effect. It has been also used as an antianxiety substance. It can be detected and quantified by using LCMS.

COCAINE AND METABOLITES

Cocaine, used for abuse purposes, is divided into two forms: (1) powdered, which can be snorted or mixed with water for injection; and (2) crack cocaine, which is not water soluble, but vaporized when heated and thus can be smoked. It lasts in the urine for a very short time (6–8 h) but produces a longer-lasting metabolite called benzoylecgonine (BZE). The author has found that EIA tests for this metabolite are quite good.

Cocaine metabolite testing using EIA at the POC can detect this cocaine metabolite in the urine for up to 3 days as it is specific for the metabolite BZE. LCMS can then be used in tandem to quantify the amount of urine cocaine or its metabolite, BZE. It can be detected in the urine of heavy cocaine users for up to 10 days.

Neither EIA nor LCMS methodology can differentiate between powdered cocaine and crack cocaine.

METHAMPHETAMINE/AMPHETAMINE AND OTHER STIMULANTS

These and other chemicals are part of the large stimulant group of substances, including ephedrine, cathinones (bath salts and flakka), MDMA (Ecstasy), Khat, MDEA, and MDA. Other chemicals such as LSD are both a stimulant and hallucinogen.

Amphetamine is a metabolite (breakdown product) of methamphetamine.

EIA testing for methamphetamine/amphetamine is known to have variable cross-reactivity with MDMA, MDEA, and MDA, so testing using this methodology is difficult to interpret as to which chemical is being detected. In addition, many medications are capable of causing false-positive results. These include Adderall, benzphetamine, bupropion, chloroquine, chlorpromazine, ephedrine, fenfluramine, labetalol, mexiletine, N-acetyl procainamide, phentermine, phenylephrine, phenylpropanolamine, propranolol, pseudoephedrine, quinacrine, selegiline, trazodone, tyramine, and Vicks inhaler.

LCMS testing will clearly differentiate amphetamine from methamphetamine. Ritalin, whose chemical structure is similar to that of methamphetamine, is an exception medication as it does not metabolize to either methamphetamine or amphetamine and has their own LCMS category (ritalinic acid).

Bath salts (cathinones, aminophenones) can be easily detected by LCMS because of their own unique molecular weight and charge.

Flakka (α-PVP—α-pyrrolidinopentiophenone), a cathinone/synthetic cocaine, which is clandestinely manufactured and very potent generator of acute psychotic behavior, can only be detected and differentiated by using LCMS methodology.

Finally, the MDMA, MDA class of stimulant substances can be detected for 1−2 days. Methamphetamines/amphetamines can be detected by EIA for 1−3 days and by LCMS for 2−4 days.

LSD, both a stimulant and hallucinogen, stays in the urine for about 2−4 days.

Nicotine can be found in the urine for about 12 h, whereas its breakdown product, cotinine, can be found for days by EIA or LCMS determination.

BENZODIAZEPINES

Benzodiazepines can be arbitrarily divided into three categories: short-, medium-, and long-acting depending on their duration of action within the body. Benzodiazepine products are difficult to interpret using EIA methodology because there are so many of them. In addition, they often cross-react poorly with existing EIA assays (e.g., lorazepam and clonazepam). Furthermore, EIA cutoff values are high, and often therapeutic amounts may not be detected when they are prescribed in low doses. Finally, medications that can cause false-positive results by EIA include oxaprozin and sertraline. LCMS technology has no problem in differentiating all benzodiazepine types and indicating their concentration in the urine sample.

LCMS technology can measure benzodiazepines in the urine as follows:

Short acting (e.g., Xanax, Ativan)—1 day.

Intermediate acting (e.g., clonazepam, Valium, Librium)—2−3 days.

Long acting (e.g., Dalmane)—7−30 days.

BARBITURATES

Barbiturates form a very large group of chemical configurations, all derived from barbituric acid, but generally classified into three groups depending on their duration of action (short-, medium-, and long-acting). Their current use is less popular than in the past.

It is interesting that most barbiturates with the exceptions of phenobarbital and butabarbital are poorly concentrated in the urine. It should be remembered that butalbital, found in combination analgesics for migraine treatment, is a noncontrolled barbiturate formulation. The only medication known to cause a false positive on the EIA phenobarbital test is phenytoin. LCMS can detect all barbiturates in the urine. Barbiturates can be found in the urine samples as follows:

Short acting (e.g., butalbital)—usually about 1−4 days.

Intermediate acting (e.g., Butisol)—40−80 h.

Long acting (e.g., phenobarbital)—at least several weeks.

Methaqualone (Quaaludes, ludes, sopers) is a synthetic barbiturate-like medication popular in the 1960s and 1970s. It can be detected in urine only by LCMS for approximately 90 h.

MARIJUANA

Marijuana comes from the hemp plant, and its principal psychoactive chemical is tetrahydro cannabinol (THC). THC concentration is highest in hash oil, which comes from the flowering tips of the unfertilized female plant, whereas hashish is lower in THC concentration.

Marijuana, like alcohol and nicotine, is considered by many to be a gateway drug, as it is thought to influence users to consider and/or try other substances of abuse.

Marijuana is stored in fat cells and thus only appears in the urine slowly. In occasional users, it is detectable in the urine by EIA for about 3 days. In chronic users, it is usually detectable in the urine for about 30−60 days and intermittently detected by LCMS, in the author's experience, in trace amounts, for up to 1 year after discontinuation. False-positive EIA tests for marijuana can be caused by the following medications: dronabinol, Sativex, efavirenz, pantoprazole, and quinacrine. CBD oil, due to its very low THC content, is usually not detected by the THC assay.

SYNTHETIC CANNABINOIDS (K2, SPICE), PHENCYCLIDINE, KRATOM, KETAMINE, AND DEXTROMETHORPHAN

Synthetic cannabinoids are a growing group of clandestinely manufactured synthetic chemicals which exhibit the effects of marijuana. However, their chemical structure is very different from that of the natural cannabinoids. Their effects are much stronger and longer lasting in comparison with the natural product. Synthetic marijuana cannot be detected in the EIA marijuana assay and can only be identified using LCMS technology for 10−12 days.

PHENCYCLIDINE, ANGEL DUST

Originally it was developed as an IV anesthetic but was never approved by the FDA because of its propensity/capability of causing amnesia, convulsions, and coma. It can easily be added to marijuana. It has analgesic and hallucinogenic properties. PCP, like marijuana, is stored in fat and other organs of the body. Thus, it can be found in the urine after a single dose by EIA testing and for the next 7 days in chronic users. LCMS is capable of finding it in the urine for even longer periods of time (up to 30 days).

KRATOM (MITRAGYNA)

Kratom is a product from plant leaves native to southern Asia. Its chemical effects are similar to those of opiates, especially morphine. It is currently legal in the United States. It is often added to tea. It appears in the urine for about 20 days and can only be detected by LCMS methodology.

Ketamine

It was originally developed as an anesthetic agent, although now is being used experimentally for depression control, PTSD, anxiety, etc.; this chemical has both sedative and hallucinogenic properties. It can be detected in the urine by LCMS for 3–4 days.

Dextromethorphan (Triple C's, DXW)

Dextromethorphan is actually a synthetic opioid which functions best in the lung as a cough suppressant, rather than for pain relief or inducing euphoria. However, at high (abuse) doses it can stimulate euphoria. It is commonly added to cough syrup. Using LCMS methodology, in people who are rapid metabolizers of this chemical, it can be detected in the urine for up to 12 h. In people who metabolize this chemical slowly, detection time increases to a couple of days.

URINE INTEGRITY, ADULTERATION AND VALIDITY TESTING

Testing for urine adulterants is one of the tools available to identify clandestine substance abuse behaviors, which the patient is trying to conceal or camouflage.

Urine testing by EIA methodology for substances at the POC is unfortunately prone to a greater amount of adulteration, tampering or providing unclear results when compared with MSMS analysis, which could potentially then have a significant impact on proper treatment and/or employment decisions. Adulteration methodology is used to "fool" this testing procedure into generating false-normal urine testing results and should not be considered valid. The way the author tries to help his colleagues understand what is happening in a nonscientific way is to have them think of an adulterant as a chemical which is able to "cover up" an EIA antibody so it can no longer attach to the substance that it is supposed to be detected. Thus, although the substance is still in the urine, it can no longer be

"found" by the antibody used by this testing method to find or detect it. The urine will now falsely appear as negative or "clean." There are a number of ways to degrade a urine sample. These are substitution, dilution, and adulteration. It also includes faulty sample collection. To try and minimize validation testing errors, the best method that the author has found is to test the patients before breakfast (in a random manner and before possible dilution from liquids ingested at breakfast can occur).

Adulterants include donated, purchased, or smuggled clean human or animal urine, available over-the-counter ingested "urine cleaner" additives to "cover up" or dilute the sample with clean urine, and certain foods or excessive fluid ingestion prior to testing will lower detectable substances to below cutoff levels, in addition to a number of easy-to-purchase common household products and newer over-the-counter drinkable masking agents which block the ability of the test antibody to bind to the substance it is supposed to detect. As noted above, adulteration can only be used to mislead initial "cup type," dipstick testing or EIA laboratory results, as LCMS testing cannot be fooled.

VALIDITY TESTING

Validity testing is an important part of testing for substances of abuse. Its purpose is to be able to alert those on the treatment team concerning possible tampering or adulteration of the urine sample.

A same-sex staff member should always be present to ensure that the urine sample is produced properly while protecting the patient's privacy and dignity when the sample is obtained. To best ensure a properly obtained sample, personal patient items should be left out of the collection area. In addition, the patient should be kept away from common bathroom items such as soap, detergent, bleach, alcohol, hand sanitizer, Visine eye drops, or ammonia in addition to other chemicals as exemplified by salt and vinegar. As noted above, newer, harder-to-detect adulterants are also now available on the open market and should be carefully watched for. Unfortunately, certain foods, vitamins, and medications can also make the urine look "strange." Finally, blue dye should be placed in the toilet and the water to the toilet be turned off during the collection period.

Hand sanitizers or other handwashing agents should only be offered after the sample has been collected and secured. After collection, the urine should be checked and noted for any unusual smell, appearance, or color by the staff member administering the test. If any of these "alterations" are found, the test may need to be repeated.

Validation testing on either presumptive or definitive testing uses the following tests:

Temperature

Creatinine

Specific gravity

pH

Oxidants

Results of these tests (except for temperature and possibly pH) can usually be found at the end of the EIA or confirmation laboratory report.

1. Temperature: Performed at the POC. Many kinds of urine test cups that can be purchased commercially have temperature testing instruments on the outside of the container. The testing should be performed within 5 min of the urine collection and be in the normal range for body temperature; otherwise this is a clear sign of possible adulteration.

2. Creatinine: A product of muscle metabolism which is produced at a relatively constant rate and excreted at that rate into the urine. A normal creatinine is above 20 mcg/mL or 20 mg/dL. If creatinine is between 5 and 20, the specimen is considered diluted (usually due to the patient drinking fluids before the test) and probably not adulterated, especially if this occurs in only one of multiple urine samples taken over time. Below 5 mcg/mL, the specimen should be considered as being potentially adulterated until proven otherwise (water is 0 mcg/mL). High creatinine levels can also result from adulterant use (they are usually very high compared with the usual normal upper creatinine reference range) or possibly suspect kidney disease if appropriate.

3. Specific gravity: Measures concentration of dissolved particles in the urine. If above 1.030 or below 1.003, suspected dilution or adulteration must be considered, unless the test is performed long after the sample has been obtained, due to normal urine changes over time. If the creatinine is also very low or high, this lends further support to the diagnosis of possible adulteration, especially if the creatinine is below 20 mg/dL.

4. pH: The pH measures acid-base ranges. If the pH is below 3.0 or above 11.0, in the author's experience, adulteration is quite possible as long as it has been checked within 5 min after the urine sample has been obtained. If both this test and the temperature are outside the expected ranges, one can be pretty sure that the sample has been adulterated or compromised, and further EIA testing of this urine sample may be considered unnecessary and obtaining another urine sample for repeat EIA or confirmatory testing should now be considered.

Please also be aware that the pH can be altered by a high-protein, low-carbohydrate diet, in addition to diabetes or a kidney/urinary tract infection.

5. Oxidants: Urine samples should be examined by the staff member present. This examination should include looking at and smelling the sample for uncommon odors, color, and other forms of unusual appearance (soapy, floating particles, cloudiness). Their presence should be noted in the patient's chart and reported to appropriate personnel.

It should be noted that the normal highest level of the reference range for oxidants is supplied by each of the manufacturers of this reagent. If a high result (above the reference range) is obtained, before serious consideration of tampering can be considered, please consider the following:

1. Check for nitrates and/or sulfates in the urine if possible, as they are oxidants whose level can increase by eating certain foods. If nitrate or sulfate levels tested are independently certified by alternative methodology and are normal, the specimen is less likely to be adulterated.

2. If the patient has symptoms of a urinary tract infection, obtain a U/A plus culture and sensitivity as urinary bacteria are capable of producing oxidants. Other "popular" adulterants include Visine eye drops and newer over-the-counter products, such as UrinAid, Klear, Whizzies, and Urine Luck.

3. Finally, high levels of the immunoglobulin (IgG [>0.5 ug/mL]) suggest adulteration with either animal urine or synthetic urine.

4. Obtain an LCMS confirmation profile because urine adulteration will only affect EIA results (the author's preferred method). Consider the adulterated EIA test as uninterpretable.

5. Another approach at this time is to watch the patient closely and repeat the test on another urine sample sometime later in the day, before obtaining an expensive confirmation profile.

---

1. Validity Testing:

   Used to ensure that the urine sample has not been tampered with or adulterated

   a. Tests include temperature, creatinine level, specific gravity, acidity (pH), and presence of oxidants

   b. Many common household or store purchased substances can cause urine adulteration

   c. Validity testing is only necessary for presumptive urine testing as confirmation testing cannot be fooled

COMMONLY USED URINE DETOXIFICATION TEST PANELS

Presumptive/screening (EIA) panel: The laboratory can perform more tests than the cup method. Please remember that not all urine cups do not test for all available substances because the cups currently available may test for anywhere from 5−13 substances depending on the antibodies present in themoops-antibody strips present in them.

1. Amphetamine
2. Barbiturate
3. BZE-cocaine
4. Benzodiazepine
5. Buprenorphine
6. Carisoprodol
7. Cotinine/tobacco
8. EtG
9. Heroin (6-MAM)
10. THC
11. Methadone
12. Methamphetamine
13. MDMA
14. Opiate
15. Oxycodone
16. PCP
17. Tramadol
18. Zolpidem

Validity Testing

1. Creatinine
2. Oxidants
3. pH
4. Specific gravity
5. Temperature

Confirmation Panel

Comprehensive: Additional tests can be added or subtracted from the detection menu when developed and/or needed.

1. 6-MAM—Heroin metabolite
2. 7-Aminoclonazepam—Intermediate-acting benzodiazepine metabolite
3. 7-Hydroxymitragynine-Kratom metabolite
4. α-OH alprazolam-Xanax—Short-acting benzodiazepine metabolite
5. α-PVP-Flakka—A cathinone-type stimulant
6. Alprazolam-Xanax—A short-acting benzodiazepine
7. AM22014OH Pentyl—A form of synthetic marijuana
8. Amitriptyline—TCA antidepressant-class sedative
9. Amphetamine—Synthetic stimulant
10. BZE—Cocaine metabolite
11. Buphedrone—Ephedrine metabolite
12. Buprenorphine-Suboxone/Subutex—A weak opiate
13. Clonazepam—An intermediate-acting benzodiazepam
14. Codeine—A naturally occurring opiate
15. Cotinine—Tobacco
16. Cyclobenzaprine—TCA antidepressant and sedative-class metabolite
17. Desmethyl cyclobenzaprine—TCA antidepressant and sedative-class metabolite
18. Desmethyldoxepin—TCA antidepressant and sedative-class metabolite
19. Desmethyl tapentadol—Opioid metabolite
20. Desmethyl tramadol—Opioid metabolite
21. Diazepam (Valium)—Long-acting benzodiazepine
22. Dihydromethysticin—Kava metabolite
23. Doxepin—TCA-class antidepressant and sedative
24. EDDP—Methadone (synthetic opioid) metabolite
25. EtG—Alcohol metabolite
26. EtS—Alcohol metabolite
27. Fentanyl—Potent synthetic opioid
28. Flunitrazepam (Rohypnol)—An intermediate-acting benzodiazepam and sedative
29. Gabapentin—Antiseizure/antianxiety medication
30. Hydrocodone—Semisynthetic opiate
31. Hydromorphone—Semisynthetic opiate
32. JWH-018-4OH pentyl, JWH-250-4OH Pentyl, JWH-073-3OH butyl-synthetic marijuana formulations
33. Kavain (Kava)—A sedative
34. Ketamine—Sedative hallucinogen
35. Lorazepam (Ativan)—Short-acting benzodiazepine
36. MDMA (Ecstasy), MDEA, MDA, MDPV—Synthetic stimulants
37. Mephedrone (4-MMC, methylcathinone)—A synthetic stimulant
38. Meprobamate—An intermediate-acting sedative, barbiturate-class medication
39. Meperadine—A synthetic opioid
40. Methadone—A synthetic opiate
41. Methamphetamine—A synthetic stimulant drug
42. Methylone (β-k MDMA, MDMA, M1)—A cathinone analogue stimulant
43. Midazolam (versed)—A short-acting benzodiazepine, sedative, and seizure prevention medication
44. Mitragynine (Kratom)—A sedative-producing chemical
45. Morphine—A natural opioid
46. Norbuprenorphine—A buprenorphine metabolite
47. Nordiazepam—A diazepam metabolite
48. Norfentanyl—A fentanyl metabolite
49. Norhydrocodone—A hydrocodone metabolite
50. Norketamine—A ketamine metabolite

51. Noroxycodone—An oxycodone metabolite
52. Oxazepam—A short- to intermediate-acting benzodiazepam
53. Oxycodone—A semisynthetic opiate
54. Oxymorphone—A semisynthetic opioid
55. PCP—An analgesic and hallucinogen
56. Phenobarbital—A long-acting barbiturate
57. Pregabalin (Lyrica)—A medication used for neuropathic pain, seizure control, and anxiety
58. Ritalinic acid—A metabolite of the stimulant Ritalin
59. Tapentadol—A synthetic opioid medication
60. Temazepam—A short-acting benzodiazepam
61. THC-COOH-tetrahydrocannabinol, marijuana, weed—A sedative-producing chemical
62. Tramadol—A synthetic opioid medication
63. Zolpidem (Ambien)—A controlled, non-benzodiazepine sleep-producing medication
64. Zolpidem-COOH-A metabolite of zolpidem
65. Extremely potent fentanyl analogues that can or have been added to standard or more specific LCMS testing menu's include, but are not limited to, the following:
    a. Acetylfentanyl
    b. AH7921
    c. Butyrfentanyl
    d. Carfentanyl
    e. Furfentanyl
    f. MT-45
    g. U-477700
    h. W-18

Addiction Management Protocols

INTRODUCTION

Pharmacologic substance abuse management for both partial or complete detoxification (more accurately known as medically supervised total abused drug withdrawal) and long-term or lifelong use of anticraving medications (e.g., naltrexone) or other forms of medication-assisted therapy (MAT) is currently available.

In actuality, however, pharmacotherapy plays only a smaller and more limited role in the entire abstinence/sobriety process. The extremely important (and actually the most critical) portion of maintaining short- and long-term sobriety is the integrated, nonpharmacologic, therapeutic approaches (e.g., mental health counseling) to assist in the lengthy brain-healing transformational changes that need to occur to allow the disordered cerebral gray matter to return to its preabuse state. Present medication therapy options are currently the only available and approved methodologies to help affected patients. Nevertheless, addiction medicine is rapidly evolving as a science with new and improved medications and psychotherapeutic treatment strategies, which are continuously being developed to further help addicted individuals successfully overcome, cure, or control this chronic medical issue. It must also be realized and taken into account that the rest of the road to long-term success (sobriety) is very individualized, and therapeutic adjustments may often need to be made to accommodate for personal variation. One example of an attempt to improve quality of care, standardization and improved treatment initiation rates and engagement of substance abuse in the recent medical literature involved the integration of clinicians and other primary care providers with additional support and training into the well-established Federal Government Healthcare Effectiveness Data and Information Set (HEDIS) quality measurement tool to evaluate performance on certain specific healthcare system measures of substance treatment options available to benefit these patients. These include improvements in identification and earlier involvement and treatment in the primary care setting and the use of age-tailored and culturally relevant demographic services by behavioral medicine specialists in addition to the focus on retention of patients in this process through the use of medication treatments.

Initial pharmacologic therapy in the author's experience, because of lack of uniform national standardization, as noted in the foreword to the book, is usually based on experience, enrollment information and team discussion, initial point-of-care urine test results and follow-up confirmations, patient admission medical condition and accompanying medications, in addition to the physical and psychiatric examinations of the patient. From this information, pharmacologic treatment can be developed and prescribed in combination with careful staff observation and monitoring. Medication type, dosage adjustment, and tapering in addition to mental health counseling gradation and treatment level are then based on patient's progress. In the author's experience, despite excellent therapy (both pharmacologic and mental health), the patients continue to feel "sick" and often take up to 18 months to feel "well or normal" again.

The object of these processes, as indicated above, is to enable the patients to gradually reduce or slowly taper and hopefully discontinue the need for one or more substance(s) of abuse in their systems on admission, under the care of a physician and the rest of the treatment team, to successfully ameliorate or stop the cravings and begin the process of long-term sobriety and thus prevent future relapse and possible overdose use of the substance(s) that they had become addicted to in the easiest, least painful, and most comfortable manner.

Almost all of our current patients present to our facility after detoxification and relapse at multiple other treatment centers. Thus, our programs include both MAT taper for opiates or their complete discontinuation and the use of anticraving medications in addition to complete detoxification to one or more of the following harmful abuse classes: alcohol, anabolic steroids, sedatives/hypnotics/anxiolytics, cannabis, cocaine, inhalants/hallucinogens/dissociatives, opioids, and stimulants.

Currently, in the author's opinion, the most difficult and frustrating component of the taper and detoxification process involves the third-party payers. This is due to the fact that many of them either fail to or simply wish not to understand that addiction is not an acute, short-term, and easily/simply treated problem, but a chronic brain disease which requires a chronic care model for treatment. Thus, they do not allow adequate time for clinically appropriate and medically necessary treatment (usually 3−5 days when up to a month may be needed) to properly detoxify and start the process to help the patient to medically and (most importantly) psychologically support his or her recovery using all required medications and nonpharmacologic available resources. This adequate time problem further continues at each lower level of care. Therefore, in the author's experience, many patients are still very sick and/or psychologically unstable when they are discharged from a detoxification level of care to a lower level of care and beyond, thus promoting a poor predicted treatment outcome and a high incidence of future drug use/relapse and possible overdose leading to death.

The way that the author has been most successful in trying to properly complete the detoxification process is to use a combination of detoxification and residential care. In both of these levels of care, controlled substances can be used as necessary and their use supervised until the process is complete or cravings are minimized or eliminated. Furthermore, additional time is available for the mental health team to maximize early psychological/psychiatric stabilization. In this way, the patients will enter the next lower level of care in a state of mind ready to engage in all necessary activities to enhance their long-term recovery process with their cravings and withdrawal symptoms markedly improved or controlled, already possibly using prescribed anticraving medications.

Furthermore, at this time, due to the early mind-clearing effects of the initial pharmacotherapy, they are also better able to participate in the crucial psychotherapy (mental health counseling) portion of the treatment process (which in the author's opinion, as previously implied, is actually the most important long-term treatment modality). In addition, the introduction of anti-craving medications at the appropriate time (see section 5) will further teach them to better deal with their addiction-related problems without the need for further detoxification treatment, in a maximally supportive, focused, and success-oriented manner, based on the specific needs of each individual patient.

OPIATES

Opiates in their natural form come from the opium poppy plant. The plant manufactures certain alkaloids, the most common being opium, morphine, codeine,

and thebaine. In fact, the United States contains 5% of the world's population but consumes more than 80% of the world's opiate supply. These alkaloids have also been modified in the laboratory to produce other formulations, the first called semisynthetic opiates. Included in this group are heroin, hydromorphone (Dilaudid), oxycodone (OxyContin and Percodan), and hydrocodone (Vicodin). Finally, opiates can be made synthetically, either legally by drug manufacturers or clandestinely in illegal laboratories. Examples of synthetic opiates include buprenorphine, methadone, tramadol, and fentanyl. Recently, extremely powerful/potent, cheap, and intense fentanyl analogue opioids (probably due to the fact that they can bind very firmly to opiate receptors) from the Far East and distributed through illegal entry into the country or the Internet have appeared on the illicit market. They have a chemical structure that differ markedly from natural opiates and thus require specialized LCMS assays for detection. These chemicals include the large animal tranquilizer, carfentanyl, acetylfentanyl, butyrylfentanyl, furanylfentanyl, AH-7921, MT-45, and W18, which are reported to be up to 10,000 times more powerful than morphine. Very likely, when used either alone or added to other substances (the process of "cutting" opiates such as heroin to make them more potent and improve the brain stimulant/pleasure effect) of abuse, it will often result in an overdose without sufficient tolerance. In fact, a simple grain of one of these substances is reported to potentially be able to cause an overdose, which can result in rapid, severe respiratory depression and/or death. Another new fentanyl-like synthetic narcotic, U-47700 has recently become more available. Called pink, pinky, or purple because of the color change from white as it is manufactured, is said to be 700% more potent than heroin. It is considered extremely powerful and dangerous. By merely touching it, a person is said to have the potential to go into cardiac arrest. The DEA has recently published a briefing guide for first responders concerning the necessary protection needed, as these fentanyl analogue opioids are also extremely dangerous to this group of law enforcement or fire department personnel who must come into contact with people who have overdosed on one of these substances. As indicated, they are extremely potent in minuscule amounts and can be absorbed into the body orally, by inhalation, and absorption through the skin or eyes.

The most deeply troubling aspect, however, is the partial or even complete reported resistance of these chemicals to the usually used doses of Narcan, the antidote for opiate overdose (possibly due to its inability to dislodge one of these newer, very powerful opiates from the receptor). Overdoses of these potent synthetic chemicals may require much larger Narcan doses (starting with 2 mg) and immediate CPR probably involving an Ambu bag (because aspiration can occur) and/or extended periods of mechanical ventilation (often days) for hopefully, successful lifesaving treatment. Please remember that a lack of oxygen to the brain for only a few minutes can cause permanent brain damage or death.

It should also be noted that heroin users have a 10%–30% higher mortality rate than users of other opiates. In addition, inhaled heroin (heroin that is heated and inhaled) use is becoming more available and popular. Its acclaim appears due to ease of administration and an increased intensity "high." Its detrimental effects are related to its enhanced brain toxicity potential.

The major effects of these chemicals are to control pain and/or generate a feeling of gratification or self-satisfaction in dependent individuals. This effect occurs for various amounts of time, which depends on the type and strength of the opiate used.

Concerning pain control, although it is difficult to quantify pain intensity, it is now well understood that opiate use should be reserved primarily for acute pain control. Furthermore, they should be used only in the minimum amount needed for adequate relief (usually 3 days but less than 1 week), prescribed for the shortest period of time of use, in addition to the concomitant use of various nonopiate pain reduction therapies mentioned previously (section 1).

Long-term opiate use for chronic pain (defined as pain lasting more than 12–36 weeks), in general, should not be considered except in special circumstances such as cancer, as its effects on pain control are usually only present for an abbreviated or limited period of time, and continued use can lead to possible addiction.

Patients using long-term opiate therapy for pain control must always be carefully monitored, and the therapeutic endpoint should not be pain control per se but improvement of impaired function and the transition to nonopiate pain relievers if possible.

It should also be noted that patients with short- or long-term hyperalgesia can also be treated with the use of MAT using methadone or buprenorphine. These latter two long-acting but weaker opiates will be further discussed shortly.

Unfortunately, and more commonly in older adults, many are prone to the pain caused by chronic medical conditions (although the author sees a large number of chronic dental problems in younger adults), often inadequately treated in the past. In these individuals the author selectively uses multiple nonopiate medications, many of which have now been shown to be non-inferior to opiates for control of moderate to severe chronic, back, hip, or knee pain over a 12-month period with fewer side effects (while continually monitoring for possible GI and cardiovascular complications), and will often require help from psychiatric and other therapy and medical specialist colleagues. In addition, other modalities such as massage, behavioral therapy, chiropractic, and acupuncture to try to control the pain as well as possible during admission with appropriate referral after discharge.

More recently, the advent of external or implanted neuromodulation or neurostimulation devices which interrupt pain signals carried by the nerves to the brain is proving helpful. In fact, CBD oil from the cannabis plant is thought to function by increasing the pain threshold, so a person will not feel the pain as intensely.

In a prone to addiction individual, who medical professionals regrettably are still unable to positively identify at this time, even innocently taking one of these potentially addicting medications in even prescribed amounts can, after only a minimal amount of time, detrimentally affect the brain when the concentration of the recently used prescribed medication (or other addictive substance) diminishes. This person will then start to become more and more dependent and begin experiencing withdrawal with all its known, increasingly negative side effects. At this time, normal life or health preservation awareness concerns, as previously indicated, start to dissolve as this individual further deteriorates into the true addiction process, which is increasingly triggered by the compulsive need for the drug in their now substance deranged central nervous systems (CNS). The only important thing in their life becomes the ceaseless search for the immediate, continually desired, persistent reuse of the craved substance despite adverse personal consequences. It is at this point that the person has fully evolved into a true substance-addicted individual.

Longer-term opiate use, even in nonprone to addiction individuals, also induces a phenomenon called "tolerance" in which larger and larger doses or more potent forms of these chemicals are required to reproduce the same "high" or painkilling effect.

Unfortunately, tolerance effects do not produce a similar consequence as it relates to the amount of opiate necessary to cause respiratory depression or breathing cessation from within the medulla of the brain, which controls automatic breathing cycles, especially the newer fentanyl-derived illicit substances. This becomes very important for those who may consume one of these extremely potent fentanyl analogues or relapse early and are actually more prone to overdose as necessary reestablishment of the "protectionary" changes in the breathing control area of the medullary part of the brain has disappeared and is no longer active.

It should be noted that NSAIDs do not act at brain opioid receptor sites.

Opiates: Short and Long Acting

Opiates can be classified in many ways. For purposes of addiction management, the author chooses to classify them in terms of their length of action (short—a few hours or long—many hours or days) and their dose per 24 h (high or low). It is also important to express that all patients who complete an opiate addiction program be given at least a prescription for a take-home overdose naloxone treatment kit to be used in case of a future overdose, either personally, if possible, or by a companion, if necessary.

Short Acting

The author has found that acute withdrawal from short-acting opioids is a 5- to 16-day process. It is usually considered to be extremely uncomfortable without pharmacologic help but usually not life-threatening.

Screening

The more seriously opioid-intoxicated patients, who often need inpatient medical attention, are usually identified on physical examination by constricted pupils, head nodding, excessive sleepiness, drooping eyelids, and track marks, while the severity of opiate withdrawal is usually classified by the author using the Clinical Opioid Withdrawal Scale (COWS), which assigns point values to 11 of the common opioid withdrawal symptoms, sweating, runny nose or tearing, anxiety/irritability restlessness, dilated pupils, current GI upset, bone and joint aches, tremor, yawning, and "goose bumps" on the skin.

Maintenance or detoxification therapy can be accomplished by substituting either longer-acting but weaker/less potent opiate methadone or the even more efficacious, partial opioid receptor stimulation medication buprenorphine (used for both complete detoxification and MAT) than the more potent opiate that the affected substance abuser has been taking. They can also be given in a dose sufficient to prevent or at least reduce the intense cravings and symptoms of withdrawal of the previously used opiate. Substitution with methadone is generally used only for long-term maintenance, starting at less than 30 mg/day, only as it is said to have a markedly diminished

potential for experiencing euphoria while eliminating the symptoms of withdrawal during the period of use. However, most of the author's patients feel that detoxification from this opiate is much more severe and longer than buprenorphine because of its slow elimination from the body (often 3—4 weeks).

Tapering and Detoxification

Complete opiate withdrawal and detoxification is most often accomplished using buprenorphine, often combined with clonidine which has proven helpful in controlling symptoms of withdrawal.

Recently, a third medication to manage opioid withdrawal has recently been approved by the FDA. It is called Lucemyra (lofexidine hydrochloride). It is intended to help mitigate the effects of opiate withdrawal but may not completely prevent them. It is a selective α-2-adrenergic receptor agonist (similar in category to clonidine), which can reduce the release of norepinephrine, said to play a role in opioid withdrawal. It is currently recommended to be used for only a 14-day period. The most common side effects reported are low blood pressure, low heart rate, sleepiness, sedation, and dizziness. The author has no experience in the use of this drug.

Finally

It should be emphasized that patients taking shorter-acting opiates cannot immediately start the withdrawal process after taking their last opiate dose.

Using buprenorphine (plain Subutex or Suboxone [Subutex plus naloxone]) or Zubsolv (similar ingredients to Suboxone) which contain an opiate blocker, to prevent IV misusage or diversion), immediately after taking the last dose of their usual opiate, will, in the author's experience, make most patients severely ill from withdrawal symptoms caused by the buprenorphine therapy itself because it is still a weak opiate.

Therefore, before starting buprenorphine therapy, they must wait till mild—moderate withdrawal symptoms begin to occur. This usually takes about 12—18 h from the time of their last dose to minimize any possible buprenorphine-induced withdrawal effects. During this time, however, they usually require medical management.

The author uses a combination of clonidine and clonazepam during this withdrawal period. These drugs have been shown to support the reduction of the somatic symptoms of withdrawal/noradrenergic overactivity, high blood pressure, and cravings (clonidine) and the often associated severe agitation manifestations (clonazepam).

Blood pressure and oxygen saturation must be regularly monitored to be sure that they are not developing severe sedation, decreased breathing (symptoms of an impending overdose), or pre- or symptomatic hypotension. (The author usually recommend that BP be taken before each dose of clonidine and not given if the BP is lower than 100/60 or the pulse rate is 55 or lower. The author further asks to be personally informed if the systolic BP < 100 or diastolic BP < 60, pulse below 55 or the patient feels or becomes faint or lightheaded before the next clonidine dose.)

The author's protocol uses 0.1 (or occasionally 0.2 mg) of clonidine and 0.5—1 mg of clonazepam tablets every 4—6 hours for opiate cravings during the 18-h waiting period.

If bedtime occurs during this period, the author uses 1 mg of clonazepam for sleep.

On awakening, if more than 4 hours are needed to reach the 18-h mark, 0.1 mg clonidine and 0.5 mg of clonazepam doses may be continued. Please remember that patients must be monitored carefully during this time and the medication dose be adjusted if necessary.

As just indicated, buprenorphine therapy is usually initiated when patients start to experience mild—moderate withdrawal symptoms. The author starts with 2 mg of buprenorphine, Subutex which is pure buprenorphine and comes in 2- and 8-mg tablets and/or Suboxone, which also must be dissolved under the tongue (the Naltrexone in Suboxone is not absorbed, just swallowed and excreted), although a 12-mg generic (Cassipa) has just been FDA approved. Subutex is preferred because of its cheaper price, as long as the patient is in a controlled environment or has experienced some sort of allergic problem/side effect to the opiate blocker portion of this medication.

If the patient feels well within 30 min to 1 hour after giving the test dose of Subutex, Suboxone, or Zubsolv (these drugs will often make them mildly ill if there is still some residual opiate left in their system), another 2 mg is given to start the tapering process. Buprenorphine or Zubsolv should be used with great caution in patients with severe asthma or significant respiratory depression, with severe hepatitis, with severe cardiac disease, and at risk for low blood pressure, and patients who are also on significant amounts of alcohol, sedatives, hypnotics, and anxiolytics, as these can enhance the depressive effects on the brain from this medication.

The tapering process is not simple for even fully committed patients as they are extremely fearful of decreasing their dose (of any substance or medication) due to their, often mistaken, belief that they will again start to withdraw and feel sick. The author usually discusses this problem at great length on admission and asks them to trust his judgment and experience. Taper also involves giving the patient only enough buprenorphine to make them feel "normal" and then slowly reducing the dose in slow increments till the patient no longer needs this medication (unless on MAT). Patients also need to be watched for stuporous or lethargic behavior in addition to medication seeking conduct. Please remember, however, that buprenorphine is still a weak but safer (lower likelihood of overdose) partial opiate formulation, which still strongly binds to opiate receptors. Once attached, it will then block the effects of other opiates; however, a patient may still experience some, hopefully mild, symptoms of withdrawal for a few days when this medication is tapered and finally stopped. In this case, the author considers Subzolv if the patient is not allergic to the naltrexone portion, as it comes in doses as low as 0.7 mg of buprenorphine.

It is important to emphasize that the initial dose of buprenorphine for any individual patient is not "written in stone" but adjusted to the needs of the person, arriving at a final dose, which will stop the cravings. Although the FDA approves higher doses of buprenorphine, 16 mg/day will fill almost all opiate receptors in the brain, so rarely more is needed unless the patient continues to have at least moderate withdrawal symptoms. The author usually starts with 2 mg, four times per day in patients on lower opiate doses but gives higher doses to those who still show withdrawal effects on this dose but rarely no higher than 16 mg. The starting dose can be adjusted up to as high as 4 mg QID or down, and the entire period of detoxification is variable depending on how the patient is progressing clinically. Because of the long half-life of this medication, the author also finds patients who prefer taking the whole daily dose one time each morning rather than the whole daily dose being given BID, TID, or QID. Finally, it usually takes the author about 10—14 days to slowly reduce the Suboxone dose to the point of complete abolishment of this drug (often due to the large amount and the extended period of time that opiates had been used before admission for detoxification), although protracted bouts of withdrawal occasionally occur, elongating the withdrawal process.

Recently, a newer buprenorphine product has been FDA approved. It is called Zubsolv. It has similar ingredients to Suboxone (as it contains an opiate blocker), but these ingredients come in additional dosage forms. The potential advantage of this medication, in the author's opinion, as previously discussed, is that during the detoxification process the use of Zubsolv can potentially enable lower doses of buprenorphine to be used so as to decrease the amount of withdrawal which may currently occur when current buprenorphine doses are already as low as possible.

When dealing with MAT, the author has found that similar to other reports, 4–8 mg of buprenorphine per day has generally been successful. The most difficult problem that the author has encountered is that patients also on benzodiazepines, alcohol, or amphetamines have often been in facilities where these drugs have been abruptly tapered and stopped before coming to our facility and must be placed back on some of these substances and then slowly withdrawn over time. The author has also needed to carefully watch these patients for medication-seeking activity or stuporous behavior in those on CNS depressants, such as clonazepam, clonidine, β-blockers, gabapentin, or muscle relaxants. Unfortunately, some use their admission for MAT to provide them with a short-term clandestine way of maintaining their former addictive behaviors by obtaining housing, meals, and medications, due to a feigned desire or personal commitment to undergo the necessary extensive mental health and other therapy modalities in addition to a fabricated long-term desire to maintain themselves on only the lower anticraving suppression doses of opiates and/or benzodiazepines.

During the early detoxification period, clonidine 0.1–0.2 mg can be used for opiate cravings, symptoms of withdrawal or anxiety, up to four times per day in addition to helping the patient with insomnia (please remember to monitor BP carefully before each dose to prevent hypotension or low pulse rate).

Comorbidities, Dual Diagnosis, and Pharmacologic Treatment Recommendations

It appears that in patients addicted to one, or a number of substances which the author is seeing more often today than in the past, it is essential to have an integrated therapy plan to treat both diagnostic domains which include psychiatric/psychological and medical problems simultaneously (dual diagnosis). Although the author leaves the treatment of complicated mental health problems to his psychiatric, medical consultant, and mental health colleagues, it is often necessary to intervene with pharmacotherapy in certain mental health and chronic medical issues before needed psychiatric, mental health, or medical consultation can be obtained. The author further considers himself lucky to have had long-term, instructive, direct interactions with his psychiatric and medical consultant colleagues, which place him in a unique position in this regard, especially in view of the fact that the mental health issues, often due to emotional stressors, often affect both the brain and internal organs such as the heart.

In older patients, one can often find more organic disease such as diabetes, hypertension, hyperlipidemia, arthritis, seizures, migraine headaches, and chronic lung disease. Sadly, both the author's younger and older patients have often been the recipients of irregular medical and dental care before admission and in need of treatment during their stay at our facility.

In addition to the psychiatric and mental health counseling, the following discussion concerns pharmacotherapy for opiate-induced comorbid disorders. However, these medications appear equally effective for similar comorbidities that may occur with the use of any abused substance or an underlying psychiatric condition.

The author's overall detoxification protocol follows the recommendations of the American Association for the Treatment of Opioid Dependence, Inc., which include appropriate safeguards to minimize problems such as using the lowest effective dose of controlled and noncontrolled medications, appropriate monitoring through urine testing, diversion prevention, various observation techniques, mental health and psychiatric treatment integration, and consideration of the use of safer alternative medications for successful detoxification and comorbidity control.

Anxiety

In the author's opinion, anxiety remains the most persistent, formidable, and challenging comorbidity encountered in a patient admitted for detoxification. It is also a major source of discussion (positive or negative) with his psychiatric colleagues. Clonazepam is the author's usual first-line, short-term choice for anxiety and can also be used for autonomic hyperactivity. (The author does not use short-acting benzodiazepines, especially Alprazolam [Xanax].) In addition, it should be remembered that most patients who enter our program may have also been using long-term benzodiazepines, either as prescribed, preadmission, or have become addicted to them through substance abuse. Thus, the challenge is to either completely taper them off this drug or slowly taper them to the lowest possible dose if on MAT, and completely and safely taper them off the use of this medication in the case of total sobriety detoxification treatment. This often takes 30 or more days to accomplish to minimize or overcome withdrawal fears, persistent withdrawal manifestations, and ameliorate long-term cravings that often continue to occur after taper, in addition to possible benzodiazepine taper resistance/opposition, especially with alcohol withdrawal. In addition, it is extremely important to remember that except for buprenorphine, methadone, or naltrexone, which may need to be used for a long period of time, only appropriate psychotherapy is the solution, and thus a major treatment priority, to fully discontinue benzodiazepine use and/or prevent future benzodiazepine relapse.

The author's protocol begins at 0.5–2 mg TID, and very slowly tapered. The author usually tapers the first half of the starting dose in no more than 0.5 mg intervals every 4–5 days. He tapers the second half of the dose slower and carefully watches for evidence of withdrawal. If this occurs, the taper is further slowed. In patients at a lower level of care, below PHP, who are employed, Valium in equivalent doses to clonazepam (5–20 mg), because of its longer clinical effect, has been successfully used on a BID dose regimen (e.g., those in a lower level of care who have started to work). Sluggish behavior should be carefully watched for, especially when initiating the use of one of these drugs, and the daily dose of these and/or other potential CNS depressant medications immediately reduced as they are a very common cause of this form of clinical response in a newly admitted, especially med-seeking patient. (However, it is often difficult to prove which medication(s) may be the cause of the problem if it occurs.) Therefore the author most often tapers the benzodiazepine dose first. However, it becomes important to investigate all of these potential depressant medications to definitively determine the cause of this problem before blaming it totally on the current dose of benzodiazepines.

It must further be strongly emphasized that there have been significant safety risks and deaths reported in addicts taking a combination of opiates and benzodiazepines. However, the FDA has recently indicated that benzodiazepines may be safely but cautiously used in patients being treated for opiate withdrawal.

The author's previous drug of choice for anxiety, which he does not routinely use currently, is gabapentin. If prescribed at another facility before admission to ours, and a specific need cannot be proven, the patient will now be slowly but totally tapered off this medication. The reason for this is because of its growing reputation as a "potentiator drug," which may enable a stronger high or "high booster" effect in combination with opiates or other abused substances. A recent study suggests that gabapentin, because of its anxiolytic, anticonvulsant, sound safety profile, and sedative properties, may also serve as a reasonable alternative to benzodiazepines if the dose of benzodiazepines becomes a safety concern, especially in the management of acute alcohol withdrawal. Otherwise, the only usual exception is for patients with proven nerve pain (with doses up to 3600 mg/day for a short period of time) or for use as an alcohol anticraving medication (900–1800 mg/day) due to naltrexone, acamprosate

failure. Lyrica, discussed below, can also be considered but is very expensive and is a controlled medication.

In view of the above, the author's present alternative drugs for anxiety control are propranolol (10–40 mg TID or QID), clonidine (0.05–2 mg TID or QID), BuSpar usually increasing up to 30 mg BID, or Vistaril 50–100 mg TID if the patient responds to one or more of them, in addition to Remeron (15–45 mg HS) due to its sleep-inducing and anxiolytic properties. Please remember that antidepressant medications also have antianxiety properties and can be very useful in combination with one or more of the aforementioned antianxiety drugs.

In the author's experience, propranolol and clonidine are fast acting and effective for acute anxiety, autonomic withdrawal symptoms, and panic attacks in addition to their use in high blood pressure (which usually takes much higher doses). They have also been helpful in controlling nightmares. Again, please be careful to monitor BP and pulse before each dose or if the patient become symptomatic for hypotension. The author will not give a dose of these medications if the BP is less than 100/60 or the pulse is 55 or below. The author only uses 0.2 mg or more of clonidine if the BP is greater than 140/100. Finally, clonidine or lofexidine (α-2 adrenergic agonists) is not recommended for alcohol or sedation hypnotic withdrawal as they mask autonomic dysregulation without improving safety.

Myopathy and Nonnerve Pain

Nonnerve pain, especially from muscle soreness or twinges, can usually be controlled with muscle relaxants (Robaxin 750 mg, Skelaxin [800 mg TID] which the author has found to be the least CNS depressing), baclofen 20 mg TID or Flexeril 4 mg TID for a short time in addition to ibuprofen or Tylenol, but the author has also had good luck with Cymbalta, meloxicam, or Voltaren and occasionally use of nortriptyline, or topical lidocaine 5% patches.

Pregabalin (Lyrica), an analogue of Lyrica, is possibly superior to gabapentin for anxiety or chronic nerve pain relief but takes about a week to work. Nevertheless, a recent report in the medical literature suggests that this medication may significantly increase the risk for opioid-related death, even on low doses versus exposure to opiates alone. It is also a controlled medication due to its addiction potential and is very expensive at this time. Thus, the author has not used it to treat his patients.

Depression

The author has found Effexor, Cymbalta, and other SNRIs and SSRIs to be effective in this frequently occurring comorbidity. However, these medications can take up to 1 month to work, and sexual side effects seem to occur fairly often. Wellbutrin XL has also been safe, even when used with other SSRIs, appears to work faster than SSRIs, promotes weight loss, and is said to have fewer sexual side effects. It may also be helpful for patients detoxing from "uppers" as it increases norepinephrine concentration (as do other SNRIs but is much less expensive) to help with the expected fatigue and has been used as a treatment for ADD and ADHD. It cannot be used in patients with an eating disorder or who are pregnant.

Finally, when using one of these medications, the patient's dose must be tapered slowly rather than abruptly stopped because neuroactive medications are capable of causing caustic withdrawal behaviors.

In addition, the author, with the supervision of his psychiatric consultants, has used Pristiq and Symbyax in patients with more severe depression (especially bipolar). These drugs work smoothly, very effectively, and quickly with fewer side effects in his experience. The author only uses Symbyax for about 1 week as it is very expensive. After that week, it is much cheaper to obtain both medications separately for continued use. Patients have not minded their weight-gaining tendencies. Other, newer medications are also available, but the author's use of them is very limited.

Finally, there has also been some success when using Prazosin 1−2 mg or Effexor (75−375 mg in divided daily doses for nightmares, PTSD, and drug dreams). However, the author's psychiatric and therapy colleagues also strongly recommend combined massed prolonged exposure therapy consisting of cognitive behavioral therapy with exposure to trauma memories.

Seizure Control

It is considered uncommon, as stated previously, for seizure activity to occur during opiate detoxification. However, in a patient who has had documented seizures in the recent past, a seizure disorder, or is on multiple substances, one or more of which are known to be associated with detoxification seizures, the author uses Keppra 500−1000 mg, two times per day or the currently preferred drug Trileptal, 300−1200 mg two times per day, which has less depression potential than Keppra and is a very helpful mood stabilizer. (Phenobarbital treatment is usually reserved for childhood seizures, but a number of addicted or med-seeking patients use this particular depressant medication not for legitimate seizure control but as a means to get a "pleasure high.")

Because the current medical literature suggests that in patients without a history of seizure activity, withdrawal seizures can occur and are most common within 1 or 2 weeks after stopping the use of these substances;

however, they have been known to occur up to 1 month later. The author uses Trileptal or Keppra for a 1-month period (while they are at our facility) in these patients and then quickly tapers and discontinues the medication. It is also important to remember that aspiration of stomach contents into the lungs can occur during a seizure, which can quickly lead to brain oxygen deprivation and resultant short- and long-term neurologic sequelae.

Attention Deficit Disorders

ADD and ADHD, arguably chronic medical problem that occurs in about 7% of adolescents and continues to increase in rate of diagnosis, in author's experience, are common complaints among patients requesting complete detoxification or MAT. It is essentially a psychiatric condition that includes hyperactivity, restlessness, and problems with attention and impulsivity management. ADHD or ADD diagnosed in childhood has been reported to persist in up to 64% of adolescents previously diagnosed and continues into adulthood in 50% of those originally diagnosed and treated as children. It is also reported that a significantly increasing number of adults use simultaneous stimulants and opioids. Furthermore, the number of children diagnosed with this disorder and who may continue to take stimulant medication continues to significantly increase. In these cases, consideration for stimulant treatment depends on the fact that the diagnosis must first be proven to have been diagnosed by a qualified health professional as a child or adolescent or within the previous 6-month predetoxification therapy. Patients with an unproven history are referred to a psychiatric colleague for diagnosis. Regrettably, a significant percentage of our patient are currently already on therapy by a physician, as these patients are often very sophisticated and use it as a way to obtain stimulant medications. Those wanting detoxification with proven ADD or ADHD may be started on replacement stimulants but may slowly be required to undergo complete taper/medication cessation (if possible). The nonmethamphetamine-derived medications for patients entering treatment found helpful by the author (and always tried first because they are not amphetamine based but certainly less successful/modest at best) are Intuniv 2−6 mg, Strattera (80−100 mg), and Wellbutrin XL (300 mg QD or BID), and Seroquel or clonidine (the latter has been used mostly in children above 6 years of age). In addition, medications such as modafinil (off-label) might be considered as they have a markedly lower dependence or possible addiction rate. Please note that these medications must be started at the lowest recommended dose and slowly be increased as recommended by the manufacturer. Finally, the long-term incidence of adverse events in those using both of these medications remains to be defined.

Mood Stabilization and Anger
In the author's experience, the drug of choice has been Trileptal. It has also been helpful with anxiety, does not require blood testing as do other medications who are bipolar, and has been extremely helpful in anger management (which has been seen most often with alcohol withdrawal). It has not been found to cause weight gain, and the patients quickly seem to feel "in better control."

Lamictal has been helpful, especially in bipolar patients in addition to other medications in this patient population. Seroquel, because of its abuse potential, increased feelings of hunger causing weight gain (especially in women), nightmares, and restless leg syndrome, has become a less popular medication except when used for insomnia or possibly schizo-affective patients. However, the author leaves the latter diagnosis to be treated by a psychiatric consultant.

Insomnia
Adequate sleep is an essential quality of life. Sleep occurs in two categories made up of five stages. The first is called non-REM (rapid eye movement) sleep, which accounts for 80% of total sleep. It occurs in four stages: two of which are light sleep, and the other two are considered deep sleep. During deep sleep, hormones are released, which are said to support immune function.

REM sleep occurs in random 90-min cycles and is thought to be vital to cognitive brain processes. During REM sleep, it is believed that the brain is able to process information through dreams, which appear to help people make sense out of life's occurrences and increase the ability to make decisions and cognitive judgments. Muscle activity is usually absent. Without the proper amount of sleep, patients are tired all day and have a difficult time functioning or participating in meaningful concurrent psychotherapy.

When choosing insomnia medications, in the author's opinion, the sleep-inducing controlled medications (e.g., Ambien) have no place in the management of detoxification. The medications found helpful by the author is Doxepin (100−300 mg), trazodone (100−300 mg), Seroquel (100−300 mg), clonidine (0.1 mg, and watch for hypotension), Remeron (15−45 mg is also very helpful for anxiety), and Rozerem, which stimulates melatonin receptors (8 mg, and again watch for hypotension), and melatonin (10 mg), a natural brain chemical, which can be purchased over the counter and can put someone into a light stage of sleep.

Psychosis
Although the management of these patients is usually left to the author's psychiatric colleagues, if needed in an urgent situation before psychiatric consultation can be obtained, Thorazine in low doses (12.5−25 mg) has been quite helpful. However, although an older medication, it has now become quite expensive. The medications most commonly used by the author's psychiatric colleagues include Abilify, Seroquel, and Latuda (which are also expensive).

Mental Health Counseling
In the author's opinion, pharmacotherapy should only be considered a short- or long-term "band-aid" (e.g., anticraving medications), whereas mental health counseling is the longer-term and most definitive treatment for continued sobriety. Mental health counseling comes in many varieties and forms and is beyond the format of this book.

Naloxone (Narcan) Treatment
Finally, the drug naloxone (Narcan), developed in the 1970s, should always be available by first responders, emergency departments, at treatment facilities or given by or to patients wherever opiate use, detoxification, or opiate maintenance treatment is taking place to reduce death from overdose. This medication, an opiate receptor blocker (μ receptors), can rapidly reverse failing respiratory/breathing or mental status function in case of an opiate overdose. It should be immediately given if the signs of an overdose are recognized (breathing problems, small or pinpoint pupils, slow heartbeat, and extreme drowsiness or you are unable to wake the person). It should also be given right away if the person is not breathing or unresponsive or even if you are not sure that the problem is due to an opiate overdose.

If possible, one should protect themselves with gloves and skin-shielding apparel due to the extreme potency and potential transferability of certain synthetic opioids, which may have been used by the unconscious victim.

After giving the medication, CPR may need to be administered till the emergency responders arrive. Withdrawal symptoms such as nausea, vomiting, diarrhea, abdominal pain, fever, weakness, tremor, and tachycardia may occur and should be expected. We have been fortunate that there has been a markedly increasing trend in the availability and use of this life-saving chemical during the last 10−15 years.

Regrettably, although this medication is reported to work in at least 90% of opiate overdoses, about 10% of those who survived the overdose do not survive a subsequent opioid overdose within the next year, possibly due to using much stronger opiate preparations. In addition, the cost of this medication has risen almost uncontrollably in the last decade, and while it can now be bought without a doctor's prescription, this fact is not well known, in addition to its markedly rising cost for unexplained reasons.

In the author's opinion, a way to think about how this chemical works is to imagine that it is able to "rip" opiates off the receptors to which it has become bound and then to cover the receptor so another opiate cannot attach to it again (while the Narcan is working). This medication can be used IV, IM, or SQ. It is also available through a handheld autoinjector or a nasal spray. Sometimes, it must also be used in conjunction with CPR for respiratory failure and/or while calling or waiting for emergency medical services.

This drug is usually given in a 0.4-mg initial dose. If there is no response within 2 min, another dose or a higher dose can be given up to 10-mg total dose. Higher doses of Narcan may need to be tried or needed during CPR and possible Ambu bag use to restore brain oxygenation for more potent or longer-acting opiates, and remember that a ventilator may need to be used—especially with the more potent opiates after lower-dose naloxone failure.

After successful use, patients must still be monitored carefully for at least 3 h because naloxone acts for only a short period of time. Thus, repeat naloxone therapy may be needed again if the naloxone effect wears off before the opiate induced respiratory suppression or depression for which it is being used (or in the case of one of the newer superpotent fentanyl analogues respiratory depression can last for a prolonged time). In this case, a ventilator may be needed for a longer period of time till the effects of the opiate wear off, which can take days.

Long-Acting Opiate Detoxification

Characterized by slower dissociation from the opiate receptor and thus a longer duration of action. Included in this group are methadone and buprenorphine. Please remember, however, that these medications only have a direct effect on opiate addiction treatment but no other abused substance. Patients on one of these long-acting opiate replacement drugs have a 70% decrease in mortality rate from a possible overdose compared with those who are not on one of these two treatment medications. They also promote improved social functioning, less criminal behavior, and reduced STD transmission.

It is also important to note that use of these medications, or complete detoxification and naltrexone use, with combined behavioral therapy, called MAT, which have been validated as effective in reducing opioid mortality, are now being considered by the Centers for Disease Control, the National Institute of Drug Abuse, and the World Health Organization as first-line therapy due to the severity of the current overdose epidemic (see the full discussion of MAT at the end of the opiate portion of this section).

Methadone Maintenence

Methadone is a synthetic opiate agonist, available as a life-saving agent since 1964, with a high fat solubility and slow metabolism. Thus, it is tightly bound to the opiate receptors for long periods of time (5−7 days). One of its most important uses is its cross-tolerance with other opiates (both natural and synthetic) so it can be used for treatment of opioid dependence by diminishing cravings and withdrawal symptoms. It can be switched with other opioids such as heroin for long-term maintenance or even detoxification or occasionally as a stand-alone opioid complete detoxification and withdrawal treatment agent. The clinical activity window for methadone is only 4−8 h although it lasts in the body for days. It is considered safe but has been known to cause overdose and death when misused. It has been shown to maintain superior retention and decreased overdose rates, plus produce better protection against fentanyl use. It is currently dispensed through only federally approved opioid treatment programs (OTPs), where patients must take the medication given, once per day (and thus inconvenient for some patients). Patients who have been in an established program for an extended period of time may be eligible to receive take home dosages.

Buprenorphine

Buprenorphine replacement, approved in 2002, can also be used for detoxification and maintenance. It is only a partial opioid agonist (and thus considered a weak opiate), longer-acting clinically than methadone and, in some patients, can be given every other day. Initial recommendations for its use indicated that a cautious approach should be used when prescribing this medication. However, after decades of research, now there are sufficient data to support a more individualized and prudent approach to its use, especially looser induction practices, occurrence of withdrawal complications, and the need for strict, continuous clinical involvement.

Physicians with special training can prescribe this medication, which can then be dispensed by a regular pharmacy. As previously discussed, it is also commonly used for detoxification and withdrawal from short-acting opiate addiction. In addition, the FDA has recently approved a longer-acting buprenorphine product called Sublocade, which the author has not used as yet. This product is injected at least once per month by a healthcare provider to ease cravings and withdrawal symptoms of opioids.

Buprenorphine is **NOT** generally considered an overdose-producing medication unless used with other depressant substances such as a rapid-acting benzodiazepine. In fact, the author has personally seen a patient with 12 buprenorphine patches on her skin, hidden under her clothing when she entered our facility. After discovery, she was only noted to be very sleepy but had no other signs or symptoms of an overdose or breathing difficulty. In addition, long-acting subcutaneous or longer-term patch buprenorphine products are currently in development.

Another advantage of buprenorphine is that it can also be used for withdrawal from methadone once the dose of methadone is reduced to the 20−30 mg/day range. In addition, buprenorphine may also be helpful in curbing cocaine withdrawal but only in high doses (16−32 mg initially and slowly tapered). Finally, in the author's opinion, the major benefit of long-term low-dose buprenorphine is because methadone is associated with a long withdrawal period (weeks to a month) before naltrexone therapy can be started. Buprenorphine will not be detected in the urine within 7−10 days and thus leaves a smaller window for relapse. However, even with buprenorphine, a patient may not wish to go through this withdrawal period and thus stay on low-dose buprenorphine, long term.

MISCELLANEOUS OPIATE PREPARATION—
Dextromethorphan (DXM), Loperamide (Imodium), Krokodil—Treat Like Other Short-Term Opiates of Detoxification

Withdrawal from methadone often takes much more time than with other opiates from 2 weeks to months. During this time, patients often remain quite symptomatic. The dose of methadone is slowly reduced/tapered by 10%−20% each day to 30 mg/day or less at which time its dose can be reduced 20% per day till complete withdrawal without continuation of serious withdrawal side effects, or to start buprenorphine detoxification treatment at that time, usually starting at 8 mg/day SL and adjusting the dose as clinically indicated. Again, buprenorphine therapy is initiated after the patient begins to have mild−moderate withdrawal symptoms from the methadone.

In the author's opinion, a fentanyl substitution patch is a usually quicker and therefore his preferred way to transition a patient using a large dose of methadone (more than 30−40 mg/day) to buprenorphine

therapy, followed by low dose (MAT level) or complete detoxification off buprenorphine and subsequent naltrexone therapy.

If the fentanyl patch is used, the daily methadone dose does not need to be changed or reduced before the fentanyl patch can be used, but only stopped on the day that the first patch is used. (Please remember that fentanyl is an extremely potent synthetic opiate and the patient can manifest increasing degrees of respiratory depression and/or stop breathing entirely.) Therefore, the patient must be carefully monitored to prevent abuse of the patch, and Narcan must be handy and the staff knowledgeable in its administration if the start of respiratory problems is detected during this 6-day period.

It is also critical that before use of the fentanyl patch, because it is a very potent opiate, one must first prove that the patient is taking methadone. These patients must be tested and be positive for methadone.

Use of a fentanyl patch is also dependent on the use of a fentanyl calculator, which can be found at http://www.globalrph.com/fentanyl.htm. The calculation is based on the daily dose of methadone. It involves using the fentanyl calculator and inserting the total daily methadone dose. The author adds an additional 25 μg/hr to the calculated dose of fentanyl.

The patches come in strengths from 25 to 300 μg/hr in 25 μg increments. The author uses the amount closest to the total fentanyl dose calculated from the methadone dose plus adding another 25 μg/hr.

Two 3-day patches will be needed to use this drug for a total of 6 days. At this time, methadone still in the patient when the process was started should be fully (or almost fully) excreted from his/her body by the sixth day of use. As noted above, each fentanyl patch should be used for 72 h. The patch should be placed on the body at 8 a.m. after the patient takes a shower and is dry. The patch is placed between the shoulder blades. After 72 h, at 8 a.m., the patch is removed, the patient takes another shower and allowed to fully dry off again. The second patch is then placed between the shoulder blades for another 72 h.

After removal of the second patch, the patient should wait till he/she starts to experience mild−moderate symptoms of withdrawal (usually about 2 h). Buprenorphine 2 mg is the given SL. If the patient feels well in the next 30−45 min, he/she should be given another 2 mg buprenorphine SL and then given 2 mg of buprenorphine TID, during that first day off the methadone patch, to start the process, and then 2 mg QID (or more if necessary) the next day. The patient must then continue the taper in the usual manner till detoxification is completed.

Clonidine and clonazepam or an alternative can also be used as needed for anxiety and withdrawal symptom control as the taper progresses, and Keppra or Trileptal can be used for those with a history of seizures. The author does not use the clonidine and clonazepam only detoxification taper.

A fentanyl patch can also be used in cases of patients using high daily doses of short-acting opiates, but only 60 h of treatment is needed. The patch can then be removed, and buprenorphine therapy can be started once mild–moderate withdrawal symptoms begin.

Finally, the detoxification protocol should offer a multivitamin with minerals because most patients admitted for various types of substance abuse have eaten poorly before admission and are vitamin and mineral depleted. Fish oil is also often recommended because the omega oils (long-chain omega 3 fats, DHA, and EPA) are said to promote antiinflammatory, brain healing, improved cognitive function, and mood stabilization by reducing inflammation. They are also recognized as important for eye, skin, and heart health plus normal immune system function. Omega oils are most commonly found in deep water fatty fish due to the fact that eat krill, or krill itself, which produce the antioxidant Astaxanthin. Omega oils can also be found in plant-based foods such as flaxseed oil.

Other important sources of antioxidants come from glutathione, which can be made from amino acids within the body but often depleted in substance abusers, and CoQ10, an important mitochondrial component necessary for energy production derived from food intake.

Finally, gut health often disrupted by substance abuse may well be improved by the use of probiotics and/or especially yoghurt.

The recent medical literature proposes that there may be a place for the use of amino acid/protein therapy to help in reestablishing the normal aggregate of the brain neurotransmitters involved in the recovery process. Those identified include tyrosine, taurine, tryptophan, D,L- phenylalanine, lecithin, and glutamate. These can be purchased over the counter at a pharmacy or health food store. The author has no experience with this therapy.

Please remember that postbuprenorphine treatment (except with the low-dose buprenorphine form of MAT) withdrawal often still occurs; however, it is usually less severe/milder because this medication is still a weak opiate, and the brain has still not had a chance to fully recuperate from its effects.

The author often uses propranolol, 20 mg, for anxiety (or sometimes more is necessary) TID or QID, as previously indicated for short-acting opiates, and/or clonidine (0.1–0.2 mg) TID or QID to help the adrenergic overactivity effects of the withdrawal process in addition to the previously mentioned medications for this purpose as listed above.

Long-Term Maintenance
The medication that the author most often uses first for this purpose is naltrexone, a long-acting, orally effective, predominantly μ-opioid antagonist, which completely blocks this receptor and thus deters the reinforcing properties of opioid (and sometimes other substances of abuse) use. It is a chemical "cousin" of the drug naloxone, the emergency drug for opiate overdose.

Further information can be found concerning anti-craving therapy in the section on long-term management of substance abuse (section 5).

MISCELLANEOUS OPIATE-LIKE SUBSTANCE TREATMENT
Kratom—A leafy psychoactive plant substance found in Southeast Asia. It has a structure similar to morphine and a morphine-like brain effect (strongly binds to opioid receptors) but is said to cause less respiratory depression. It can be chewed or is added or made into tea. A recent FDA statement underscores its potential for abuse and should not be used to treat a medical condition or as an alternative to prescription opioids, as there is no clear evidence for any medical use of this substance. Finally, its use has resulted in multiple FDA-reported deaths. It is still legal in the United States. Treat as a short-acting opiate if necessary as recent reports indicate that buprenorphine and naltrexone have been effective. Finally, dextromethorphan (DXM, a cough suppressant) and loperamide (Imodium), a medication to slow bowel motility, are both opiate class medications, which work on opiate receptors outside the CNS. If used in dosages, which exceed those recommended, an opiate-like anesthetic reaction often occurs. The effect is usually short acting (hours).

Krokodil (crocodile)—Originated in Russia from a codeine base, which is available over the counter in that country. This drug has been spreading across Europe. It is said to "eat junkies alive" because it can cause disfiguring green-black skin, gangrene, and scaling secondary to infection from some of the ingredients that are mixed with the codeine.

MEDICATION-ASSISTED TREATMENT
Overview
MAT for long-term maintenance management of patients addicted to opioids, although still markedly underused, has recently reemerged as an important

tool or way to normalize brain chemistry and prevent or reduce fatal overdoses and thus save lives. This concept originally came into existence as a federally sponsored methadone treatment program, which is still available today. However, with the later development and employment of the drugs such as buprenorphine, a partial opiate agonist (methadone is a full, but weaker agonist) which is also considered useful, but a much more toxic drug and less available as it can only be distributed from certain designated centers, for detoxification or maintenance treatment of opiate addiction, and the development of naltrexone, the opioid antagonist, anticraving medication, an increasing trend toward long-term maintenance, after partial detoxification using buprenorphine, or full detoxification and the subsequent use of naltrexone, began to emerge.

However, because of a pronounced increase in the incidence of opiate relapse and overdose in recently fully detoxified patients who did not choose to begin MAT therapy (within the first 6 months of detoxification), in comparison with those who continue to use opiates without detoxification, combined with the often associated increase in the severity of continued comorbidities (especially anxiety and depression) after total detoxification completion, and the associated markedly enhanced fatal outcome potential (from respiratory depression or paralysis during an overdose, or suicide from a nontreated or incompletely treated psychiatric comorbidity), a reassessment study of postadmission maintenance therapy using either long-term liquid methadone (30 or less mg/day) or more often, low-dose, partial detoxification, sublingual buprenorphine (4–8 mg/day) or postdetoxification naltrexone treatment was advocated and the results carefully studied. The recommendation is to use these medications as long as benefits continue to be provided.

Based on these studies, it has now been conclusively demonstrated that, when used in a safe medical setting, at prescribed doses, in conjunction with simultaneous behavioral therapy, counseling and possible targeted brain stimulation treatment, psychiatric comorbidity medication management, there are now more useful, long-term alternative techniques, which have the potential to eliminate sedation, cravings, and the negative effects of short-acting drugs of abuse by blocking the craving effects of opiates, so they have no more desire to use opiates or respond to time, place, or person environmental cues, which are known to stimulate the cravings that can result in possible relapse and/or overdose.

Furthermore, based on multiple evidence-based studies, these therapeutic modalities do not appear to possess the same potential to make the users "high" or produce craving behaviors as seen with high-dose

opiates. In fact, they have the opposite effects as these "safer" opiate medications occupy but do not stimulate the receptors that produce this phenomenon, plus the use of additional comorbidity medications, brain stimulation, and nonpharmacologic psychotherapeutic techniques, which appear to be able to modify or erase the effect of environmental craving producing stimuli for which addicted individuals can relapse.

Although long-term confirmatory data are still lacking, MAT appears to provide a very beneficial form of longer-term maintenance, available for those addicted to opiates, which will allow them again focus, improve learning, and thus enable them to make sound and complex judgments, regain control of their lives, to begin a fresh, more reasonable, responsible, productive normal life as nonaddicted individuals: in essence, keeping them alive as they continue to work toward and then maintain sobriety. Success of this management option has now allowed recovered individuals to become valuable role models for those not yet at this stage of rehabilitation, similar to people with other chronic conditions, without the previous negative stigma of an individual just "substituting one addictive substance for another," which as previously mentioned is simply not true because these medications will only produce dependence so as to prevent other opiates from occupying brain opiate receptors, rather than true addiction which is defined as the overwhelming brain compulsion for continued substance use coupled with total disregard for self-harm caused by the unremitting use of these chemicals.

MAT maintenance has also demonstrated the ability to deter the probability of future opiate abuse, continuation of current illegal or deviant social behavior, and a marked decrease in the transmission of infectious diseases.

Although MAT treatment can be initiated using methadone, naltrexone, or buprenorphine, the latter medication, which is considered a much milder and safer opiate, with shorter and less severe withdrawal symptoms compared with methadone, is why this medication appears to be the most ideal for MAT at this time.

This drug, when administered long term, has been shown to significantly reduce mortality and morbidity (e.g., overdose potential, prolonged withdrawal symptoms, and relapse) in patients originally addicted to other forms of opiates. In fact, recent FDA statistics indicate that MAT therapy has decreased the overall risk of death from all causes by half. Thus, patients can now initiate MAT, consisting of a taper to a small amount of daily or every other day buprenorphine, weekly patches, or the recently FDA-approved 1-month long-acting buprenorphine implants called Sublocade or naltrexone so as to be able to function completely normally in society and the workplace on a daily basis.

In the author's opinion, the major benefit of using buprenorphine rather than methadone is because the use of naltrexone, either short or long acting, requires that the patient be completely free of opiates before initiation of this drug, which many patients choose not to want to do because stopping opiates for 7—10 days using buprenorphine or up to 1 month for methadone will certainly cause withdrawal problems.

MAT medications have other important advantages as they can also be helpful in ameliorating pain. As you may know, many opiate users originally used more potent, prescribed opiates for pain control, but then became addicted by overuse, subversion, or tolerance of one of these medications, rather than being placed on them **only** in the recommended low dose and short time frame (3 days or definitely less than 1 week). This recommendation also applies to both the use of more potent opiate in addition to one of the underprescribed and/or underused MAT medications. In addition, easily available, over-the-counter (OTC), nonopioid pain-relieving preparations have now been shown to have the same long-term benefits as opiates for certain types of noncancer pain control and should be seriously considered (see above).

The growing pain control use of opiates to the initiation of an opiate addiction problem is often due to the fact that many prescribing physicians inadvertently and unfortunately play an enabling role in this problem. This is often due to lack of training in this area of medicine, understanding that these opiate preparations are capable of initiation of opiate desires in as short as 1 day and increasing with time, especially in addiction-prone individuals. There is also lack of confidence, especially in the benefits of buprenorphine, whose advantages easily outweigh its possible addiction risk, inadequate basic knowledge about this medication, or failure to obtain the required FDA-prescribing certification (which only a very small percentage of opiate prescribers have). Finally, buprenorphine, or naltrexone, as opposed to methadone, also has the advantage of being available by prescription through most pharmacies.

In summary, the best comments supporting the use of MAT for expanding the use of this lifesaving treatment have been made by the FDA Commissioner, Scott Gottlieb.

His comments may be summarized as follows.

Unfortunately, far too few people who are addicted to opiates are offered an adequate chance for treatment that uses medications, often due to inadequate insurance coverage. In his report, he also cited a Massachusetts report indicating that 1.1% of those who started methadone or buprenorphine after a nonfatal overdose compared with 2.3% of those who did not receive treatment—a risk reduction of more than 50%.

In addition, he drew the distinction between addiction to and a physical dependence on opioids. "Addiction involves continued use despite harmful consequences and psychological craving beyond physical dependence but noted that someone who is physically dependent on opiates without craving more or harming themselves or others is not addicted."

OUR PROTOCOL

Our protocol is a similar three-step process, which is contained in the previously discussed US Department of Health and Human Services protocol for comprehensive drug treatment or detoxification and the recent medical literature guidelines. It again includes evaluation, stabilization, patient documentation, and tracking plus helping place currently dependent, but highly treatment success motivated patients into an appropriate level of care to initiate their long-term treatment program.

1. **Evaluation**

The key to our evaluation process is to understand the motivation for treatment of any person who wishes to enter our program. We are only interested in accepting those who are committed to long-term full detoxification sobriety or lifelong MAT and not to use our facility for their own selfish benefit of obtaining substances and temporary housing (a short-term roof over their head, healthy meals, and the ability to legally obtain controlled medications while there). Our screening and evaluation process is very extensive, complex (although not perfect), and we are very explicit and up-front with our expectations because many of our patients think that because they will stay on buprenorphine or naltrexone, that they will not be expected to greatly taper other substances such as benzodiazepines.

When evaluating our patients, pretherapy, we are indeed fortunate to have both experienced, highly trained mental health counselors and a PhD-level psychologist to interview and evaluate them.

In addition, those accepted are carefully watched for both signs of noncompliance with the elements of the program or especially drug-seeking behaviors (the achievement of a short-term clandestine way of maintaining their former addictive substance habit and obtain housing due to a convincing but fraudulent strategy to persuade us that they plan to comply with the principles of the program). In addition, hiding substances of abuse on their person, their belongings, or in body cavities on admission or finding a way to obtain them after admission, plus unreported mental health issues that need to be addressed with our treatment team and corrected before a successful outcome can be achieved.

During the evaluation process, prospective patients, many of whom are currently on multiple substances of abuse, often in large amounts for many years, must agree to our goal of substance tapering and nonpharmacologic brain stimulation techniques. This process is undertaken with the hope of significantly reducing or hopefully terminating the use of all these substances with a concurrent reduction in the buprenorphine dose to a level which prevents opiate cravings (usually 4–8 mg/day) or total detoxification and naltrexone use which allows for normal daily functioning. In fact, patients who are admitted after relapse should not be denied buprenorphine treatment in addition to other necessary resources and traditional mental health counseling support.

In our experience, complete termination of benzodiazepine usage is often difficult to accomplish, although always being vigorously attempted. The author and his psychiatric colleagues are continually being caught in the conflict of potentially placing the patient at risk for further substance abuse by continuing to prescribe this medication versus failing to provide adequate treatment during withdrawal (especially due to the lengthy time needed to successfully withdraw from benzodiazepines, as many patients have taken benzodiazepines for years at prescribed doses before admission). The effect of this continuous conundrum usually results in the careful but necessary use of benzodiazepines, especially early in MAT treatment or for continuation of benzodiazepines (with the exception of alprazolam, which is more frequently involved with overdose) after a short detoxification to prevent possible seizure, and minimize withdrawal symptoms, but then slowly being tapered as close to or preferably complete termination, as possible. In fact, due to the fact that buprenorphine is only a partial opiate, research into coprescribing buprenorphine and benzodiazepines has not been associated with a large number of postmortem toxicology reports (it is most commonly found with IV benzodiazepine and alcohol use). Nevertheless, please remember that even after successful benzodiazepine detoxification, one should expect a number of days when mild–moderate withdrawal symptoms will occur. Antiseizure medication should be continued at least while the benzodiazepine withdrawal effects continue to persist. However, if the clinical necessity to use benzodiazepines remains (e.g., a difficult to control panic disorder before a prescribed antidepressant starts to work successfully), the patient may continue taking a low dose of this medication at discharge (usually 1 mg or less of clonazepam, two to three times per day at our facility). This is permitted in the FDA, MAT guidelines.

Another evaluation goal is to help the patients understand the benefits and potential problems associated with this type of program that this is a long-term process and that they may need to stay in our facilities at different levels of care for months at a time or more than the usual 30-day treatment and taper program.

Finally, our patients need to become aware of the fact that achieving the goals of our program may involve some discomfort or pain but that the ends will justify the means as they slowly regain their self-esteem, decision control making capabilities, and finally earn their rightful and desired productive place back in society.

2. **Stabilization and medication taper**

At this time, although the principles of MAT are quite sound in theory and well documented statistically, long-term treatment of opiate addiction using buprenorphine or naltrexone still lacks abundant practical experience and standardization. Our program, as previously indicated, stresses a 30-day program consisting of daily meetings with the clinical staff and at least once per week discussion with the medical director to discuss patient problems and successes, medication taper, and using evidence-based technologies including targeted brain stimulation techniques and intuition to perform best practice medicine and mental health counseling, as drug-seeking behaviors are the most difficult challenges to the stabilization process and best treated long term with continuous psychological counseling.

In our facility, the percentage of med/substance-seeking patients who we interview has appeared to increase since we started the program. Some of these patients have become very sophisticated (often by contacting one or more of the patients currently or previously in the program) and often have actually entered the program through deceit. Luckily, we have become increasingly skilled in detecting their medication-seeking behavior or intentionally omitted or unknown mental health issues. Additionally, once some of these patients are placed on even reasonable tapered starting doses of these previously used substances, it sometimes becomes both very frustrating and difficult to taper the dose to the recommended final expected amount as these patients are very fearful of symptoms of withdrawal. Thus, we have found that participants in our program must first agree to start on no more than

8–12 mg of Subutex and 1–1.5 mg of clonazepam (however, modifications of these doses can occur based on patient fear or signs of withdrawal). Once mental health counseling takes hold, taper becomes easier. In addition, we do not use methadone in our program.

Patients who balk at our substance limits, unless there is a proven reason for higher medication doses on admission, are then be offered the alternatives of staying in our program and "playing by our rules or face discharge to an alternative program."

Patients who enter our program are first taught to understand that our goal is primarily to save lives by preventing relapse and overdose. Therefore, before placing them on any controlled medications (except for buprenorphine), they must supply us with proof of previous physician prescription or urine test confirmation. Once the need for one of these medications has been established, they will initially be continued on their formerly abused, controlled substance(s) up to their preadmission doses if absolutely necessary. They may also need be started on proven alternative medications known to prevent potential life-threatening side effects if one or more previously used regulated medication must be discontinued. These substances or alternative medications will then be slowly tapered during our 30-day medication management or total medication withdrawal period, to prevent the serious side effects from a rapid taper, especially substances known to cause seizures from a precipitous taper or immediate discontinuation (e.g., alcohol, benzodiazepines, amphetamines). Our program also encourages tapering off gabapentin and other unnecessary sedation-producing medications in addition to appropriate professional consultation, mental health therapy, and use of community resources.

Again, it must be remembered that, in our program, the time needed to taper a patient from a controlled medication is not written "in stone" as often done in other complete detoxification or other MAT programs. Thus, the short duration usually specified by an insurer is often inadequate to complete our role of slowly decreasing/tapering or weaning the patient from a large dose of a pretreatment-controlled drug or abused substance so as to minimally predispose them to the effects of withdrawal, relapse, overdose, and possible demise.

The reason for the slow taper is to remember that substance-addicted brains have been chemically and anatomically altered from their normal state to one with a new homeostasis point. Healing should thus be considered a similarly lengthy or even lifelong process, which we are just beginning to understand.

Furthermore, the length of the detoxification or substance reduction process is often different for most abused substances and also depends on the metabolic rate of each addicted individual (e.g., shorter for opiates and longer for benzodiazepines and amphetamines). Although our program has detoxification protocols for each abused substance, the amount of substance previously used and length of time used must also be taken into consideration.

Our stabilization program also includes random urine drug testing, blood wellness testing (if not recently performed) to better understand the current condition of their organs, and STD evaluations plus pregnancy testing in female patients. Our patients can then be offered appropriate treatment for their often previously untreated medical or mental health problems by our medical director and counseling staff.

Included also is instruction in smoking cessation, use of long-term medications to prevent cravings, complete detoxification if requested, STD counseling in addition to properly learning and taking part in activities of daily living, clean housing, nutritious and healthy meal planning, and cooking. Furthermore, other services that can include a combination of the following helpful essential family, educational, social, workplace, and community reconciliation strategies are as follows: massage, acupuncture, chiropractic, aerobic exercise, yoga, palates, spiritual guidance, attendance at alcoholics anonymous or similar organizational meetings, and short- and long-term-linked cognitive/behavior modification/psychological/psychiatric strategies and targeted brain stimulation to minimize or eliminate biological and/or environmental craving clues.

3. **Appropriate Level of Care Placement**

Not all of our patients who come to our program are admitted to the same level of care. In addition, their time spent at any particular level of care is variable and based on individual progress, until they finally reach the level of complete independence. The initial level of care is determined by our evaluation team and depends on many factors including their level of understanding, previous experience, amount and length of substance abuse, formal education, and mental health handicaps or concerns.

During their time in our facility, they are reeducated as previously noted in activities of daily living and self-care including chores and active participation in group activities to help with self-esteem recovery.

Finally, after program completion, especially in view of the fact that many of our patients are not residents who live in the immediate area of our facility, we spend a great deal of time and effort to find them the proper healthcare team who not only understands MAT but are also fully staffed to continue the comprehensive process initiated in our facility. Finally, we are interested in long-term feedback to quantify their progress and provide our program with additional input and success statistics. Part of this feedback involves the importance of placement into housing that promotes continuation of sobriety and avoidance of craving-associated situations or temptations.

In conclusion, we believe our program is somewhat unique in that it is state of the art, has a noble mission, and is available to anyone committed to breaking the cycle of substance abuse, addiction, relapse, and overdose. Use of this treatment program will hopefully permit their return to society in a nonstigmatized, healthy, and productive way. This also includes the fact that patients using MAT for long-term or lifelong opiate abuse control are protected under the Federal "Americans with Disabilities" nondiscrimination laws to aid them in their return to society (e.g., employment and housing).

ADDICTION MANAGEMENT PROTOCOL-ALCOHOL

Introduction

Alcohol is a CNS depressant and is known to add to the similar effects of other CNS-acting substances when used together. Alcohol use disorder (AUD) is reported to cause 88,000 deaths in the United States annually in addition to its high continued use morbidity (clinically significant impairment leading to a mediocre quality of life) usually from severe liver disease (cirrhosis) or liver cancer. It is said to affect 14% of our population, but only about 8% seek treatment. It still remains the drug of choice for college students and makes a person more prone to depression. DSM-5 contains a full diagnostic classification of AUD. Teenage users have been shown to have an increase in short- and long-term cognitive problems. Long-term use can lead to one or more psychiatric comorbidities, including PTSD, psychosis, and worsening of schizophrenia manifestations. Death usually occurs during precipitant withdrawal. Because of its legal status, abuse often starts in the teenage years.

Women absorb alcohol faster than men. Thus, they commonly reach the legal limit after only one drink, whereas it takes two for most men under 65 and one drink for men over that age (a "standard" drink is considered 0.6 fluid ounces of alcohol or 12 ounces of beer, 5 ounces of wine, or 1.5 ounces of hard liquor). This also translates to 196 g of pure alcohol (11 glasses of wine or beer) per week for men and 98 g of alcohol per week for women.

The US Preventive Task Force (USPSTF) recommends the following:
1. Healthy adult men, aged 21—64 years, should not drink more than 4 drinks per day or 14 drinks per week.
2. Healthy men aged 65 years or older should not drink more than three drinks per day or seven drinks per week.
3. Healthy women of all ages should not drink more than three drinks per day or seven drinks per week.

Obviously, although these guidelines are a good general recommendation, many drinks obtained at parties, taverns, or restaurants contain either a greater or lower concentration of alcohol found in one of their "standard" drinks.

A comprehensive, recent study has further recommended lowering the threshold for lowest all-cause mortality. This involves no more than 100 g of pure alcohol per week (5 drinks per week) expressed as a 1—2 year longer life span (decreased stroke, heart failure, aortic aneurisms, heart failure, and fatal hypertensive disease) in people who drink the lesser weekly amount. Binge drinking, classified as more than five drinks on the same occasion for men and more than four drinks for women, is also on the rise, especially in the elderly, and lifelong drinkers experience increasing frontal lobe deficits. Finally, heavy alcohol use is defined as binge drinking on more than 5 days per week.

Alcohol, which increases dopamine concentration through its effects on the GABA and NDMA receptors in the brain, is one of the most common reasons for admission to a detoxification unit. It is metabolized and secreted into the urine at a constant rate (about 20 mg/dl/h) independent of the amount ingested. Chronic alcohol toxicity can damage the brain, both acutely or long term, including the increased risk of future dementia. It can also cause somatic medical problems such as liver and heart disease; contribute to the incidence of hypertension, type 1 diabetes, and stroke; and is capable of influencing the occurrence of a number of cancer types. In fact, even modest alcohol ingestion has been implicated in limited improvement in nonalcoholic fatty liver disease and significantly lowering the odds of resolution of nonalcoholic steatohepatitis. It can also affect fetal growth and development and accounts for one-third of all motor vehicle fatalities. Small amounts each day are still considered beneficial, especially red wine (one drink or less for women and two drinks or less for men). Fifty percent of AUD risk is thought to be transmissible by a genetic predisposition, and 50% appears attributable to environmental factors such as various forms of child, adolescent, or household instability, the effect of the many diverse life stressors and/or abusive behaviors. Depression appears to increase alcohol relapse in women but not men, and risky/unhealthy drinking behavior has been associated with symptoms of PTSD.

The author's treatment guidelines in primary care settings for this condition are as follows.

Screening

1. Patients (adults 18 years of age and older in addition to pregnant women) should be screened for unhealthy alcohol use or more than the recommended daily or weekly amount of alcohol (AUD) at each visit to a healthcare provider. Although the evidence is still insufficient in teens, 12–18 years of age, screening is still a good and prudent practice. Positive results should result in referral for behavioral counseling to promote habit change. Although a number of brief questionnaires exist for the primary care setting (e.g., AUDIT-C, SASQ, CAGE), the author, who only sees patients with an already confirmed diagnosis of dependent or addicted behavior, uses the Clinical Institute Withdrawal Assessment-Modified (CIWA) Alcohol scale in which a high score should trigger the need for detoxification or stabilization, rather than just counseling; it consists of an evaluation of the following signs and symptoms: nausea/vomiting on evaluation, tremors, sweating, anxiety, sensory clouding, agitation, skin sensory changes, visual disturbances, headaches, elevated BP, or pulse.

2. If severe alcohol use or risk of AUD is suspected, the need for inpatient detoxification or stabilization should be addressed. If mild–moderate AUD is suspected, counseling and possible intensive psychosocial intervention referral should be suggested, and possible medication therapy should be discussed, hopefully accepted, and then prescribed by the treating physician.

3. Before admission to a detoxification treatment facility is considered, it is imperative that the patient be screened for severe inebriation, including an EKG to assess the length of the QT interval for prolongation as it may identify a life-threatening ventricular arrhythmia (Torsades de pointes, TdP) or point toward cirrhotic cardiomyopathy and/or disease severity, for which a preadmission, short hospitalization may be required.

4. Treatment of alcohol addiction uses Narcan treatment for respiratory distress in addition to a number

of drugs for the different problems faced by alcoholics during withdrawal.

a. Hepatic encephalopathy

Because the liver plays an important role in detoxification of harmful chemicals from the intestinal tract, hepatocellular dysfunction can result in both cognitive and psychomotor impairment. Although bleeding into the intestinal tract is a well-described cause of this type of cerebral impairment, one of the common reasons for this problem is an alcohol-induced, liver-impaired detoxification problem due to the increased levels of blood ammonia rather than ammonium levels (due to ammonia production from gut bacterial or fungal overgrowth metabolism from alcohol-induced stomach mucosal damage) which can become injurious to CNS function.

A simple measurement of this chemical (ammonia) is advised for all patients admitted for alcoholism, especially those who already exhibit signs of cognitive deficit, hand tremor, or asterixis (liver flap). Elevated levels of ammonia in the blood can be treated with lactulose and/or antibiotics. Lactulose is digested by colonic bacteria and results in colon acidification forming ammonium ion rather than ammonia. Ammonium ion is nonabsorbable from the gut and thus not able to produce potential CNS neurotoxicity.

The author initially uses 30 mL of lactulose three to four times per day. Ammonia levels should be followed serially, and the dose of lactulose should be titrated so two to three soft daily stools are produced.

In patients who are unable to take oral medication, rectal lactulose may be indicated. The dose is 300 mL of lactulose in 700 mg of saline or sorbitol as a retention enema for 30–60 min. This can be repeated every 4–6 h.

Oral antibiotics have also been used successfully to control ammonia-producing gut bacteria and can be used with lactulose, but this form of therapy is beyond the scope of this monograph.

b. Seizure prevention and anxiety control

In alcoholics who have recently been drinking, the author has found that they often arrive for admission with moderate symptoms of acute intoxication or withdrawal, especially neurologic symptoms including loss of muscle coordination, mental impairment, ataxia, nausea, and vomiting. Although the intermediate-acting benzodiazepine clonazepam, 0.5–1 mg TID or

QID in mild acute alcohol withdrawal is most often used and preferred because of its smoother clinical course, the shorter-acting benzodiazepine, rapid-acting Ativan (lorazepam) 1–2 mg, four times per day PO may also be considered, in addition to the intermediate-acting benzodiazepam Librium (chlordiazepoxide) 25 mg QID or the longer-acting Valium (5–10 mg TID), also have been used for both potential seizure protection and cooccurring, acute anxiety and sedation problems during detoxification. These medications can be tapered (TID, BID, QD, half-QD) as clinical conditions improve. Remember, however, that benzodiazepines must be used with caution in certain populations such as older adults and those with liver dysfunction. In addition, Keppra or Trileptal BID for 30 days is also prescribed for additional seizure control, especially in patients who have had seizures in the past or those who have completed a short-term detoxification program and are now being treated at a lower level of care where benzodiazepines are no longer being prescribed. Finally, after slowly tapering benzodiazepines, anxiety control is usually continued with buspirone (BuSpar), 15 mg QID or 20 mg TID, propranolol TID or QID (with proper BP and pulse monitoring). Clonidine is not recommended in alcohol detoxification. See anxiety control in opiate portion of this section.

Another useful medication, if absolutely necessary (see section on opiates) for both seizure control and craving cessation, and anxiety is the GABA agonist Neurontin (gabapentin), 300–600 mg TID. Please again remember that this medication has an abuse potential when used in high doses, especially in adolescents and young adults. Tachycardia and seizures are also implicated.

Additional Treatment Strategies

Muscle relaxants and NSAIDs are helpful for muscle aches or twitches, which are common during alcohol withdrawal.

Depression is also frequently temporarily seen. The antidepressants mentioned in the opiate section are quite successful in addition to psychotherapy.

Trileptal, as noted in the opiate section of this chapter, has been very helpful to ameliorate the often seen disrupted social cognition (expressions of anger) during detoxification in addition to its seizure prevention capabilities.

1. There are multiple medications for the treatment of alcohol cravings as they are said to modify motivation to use ethanol. See section on long-term medication options to help curb substance abuse. Of these, three are approved by the FDA (naltrexone, acamprosate [Campral], and disulfiram [Antabuse]. Baclofen, gabapentin, and topiramate (Topamax) are also commonly used "off-label." Lyrica and Chantix may also have this potential.
2. Other, sometimes helpful, OTC medications include the following:
   i. Mega B vitamins
   ii. Vitamin C
   iii. Multivitamins with minerals
   iv. GABA-600 mg PO TID
   v. CoQ10
   vi Fish oil
   Alcohol use patients are often vitamin B and C depleted as these are water-soluble vitamins (and they urinate a lot). These supplements are usually given for at least 1 month. GABA is sold over the counter and will fill up the same receptor sites that alcohol uses. Fish oil is helpful for CNS inflammation.
3. Chantix for smoking cessation and gabapentin have now been approved by the American Psychiatric Association for alcohol-craving cessation if naltrexone and/or acamprosate fail. Please remember that Chantix appears to work at the sites of the addiction pathways of the brain, so that these patients may not only stop smoking but in addition, Chantix may help in the same way for other forms of compulsive or substance abuse behaviors. Please remember, however, that Chantix can produce severe depression and/or suicidal thoughts in a minority of patients so they must be carefully monitored. Gabapentin misuse, it should be remembered, is capable of producing serious withdrawal effects and documented demise.
4. Finally, recent research reports indicate that drinking a few cups of coffee each day may be helpful in repairing alcoholic liver damage (in addition to helping migraine headaches).

ADDICTION MANAGEMENT PROTOCOLS—COCAINE, AMPHETAMINES, AND OTHER STIMULANTS

Introduction

Stimulant drugs induce elevated catecholamine levels, plus enhanced neurotransmitter activity including dopamine and serotonin. Cocaine is often snorted in its salt form, but in its freebase form, called crack cocaine, it is smoked. Chronic cocaine and amphetamine usage is often associated with cognitive impairment, psychiatric and neurologic disorders (similar to traumatic brain injuries). Chronic amphetamine and methamphetamine usage is also associated with increased seizure activity and can induce a psychotic state that may be long-lasting or recur after apparent detoxification. IV amphetamine use is capable of causing an inordinate loss of brain function. In the author's experience, acute cocaine effects are usually just "slept off." Habitual cocaine use, however, is a frequent cause of nasal destruction and deviated septum. Long-term stimulant usage can affect not only the brain but also the heart, lungs, sexual function, and the kidney. Psychostimulant drug withdrawal may often promote severe depression.

Unfortunately, the treatment of stimulant drugs is considered "uncharted territory" as there are no satisfactory, established, effective, FDA-approved medications for detoxification from this class of chemicals. Thus, the treatment used is a combination of the current sparse medical literature plus the author's experience.

The author usually considers stimulant drug formulations to be made up of three loose categories: cocaine, methamphetamine, and others. Treatment for all groups are somewhat similar with the object being to get the patient to relax and minimize agitation while reducing autonomic stress on all effected organs till the substance(s) have been cleared from the brain and body and to start them back using a healthy meal plan for the often seen weight loss or malnutrition.

Treatment

1. **Cocaine abuse**
Evaluate patient for severe arrhythmia, chest pain possibly leading to an MI, suicidal ideation, or depression during the first week of withdrawal as it may require a short hospitalization. In author's experience, however, the great majority of patients are at lower risk as they are more likely to fall asleep after using this drug and "sleep it off as previously indicated." However, use Keppra or Trileptal for seizure prevention. Moreover, the current medical literature indicates that these medications may play a role in reducing cravings.

Baclofen—This medication has been found to be helpful with cravings and to relax muscles. However, some studies have not found this medication to be useful in cocaine withdrawal. Its results have been variable in cocaine-addicted patients in author's experience.

β-Blockers—atenolol 25−50 mg can be used with caution to protect the heart as long as no contraindications exist. Monitor blood pressure and pulse rate carefully to prevent hypotension. The medical director or on-call physician or nurse should be called if necessary.

Modafinil, 100−200 mg PO, QD, or BID (8 a.m. and 12 p.m.) for at least 2 weeks to suppress or substitute for stimulant intoxication from previously used high doses of cocaine. Please note that this medication is very expensive in the nongeneric form, and insurance companies do not like to authorize its use for any indication beyond that approved by the FDA. It is also a low-level controlled medication with decreased potential addictive properties.

Desipramine, 150−300 mg has been successfully used for this purpose.

Naltrexone 50 mg. PO daily, providing the patient is clear of opiates.

Short-acting benzodiazepines (Ativan, 1−2 mg TID-QID) or clonazepam 0.5−2 mg TID or QID for agitation if necessary.

Wellbutrin XL, which also inhibits norepinephrine reuptake to help the often seen fatigue in these patients, has been the preferred initial antidepressant.

Doxepin, 100−200 mg. H.S. for sleep as needed. It also decreases norepinephrine reuptake.

Dopamine agonists: bromocriptine, pergolide, and amantadine have been used to increase dopamine production and thus ameliorate the systemic effects of cocaine. The author, however, has little experience with these medications.

Buprenorphine in doses of 16−32 mg (but not lower) has also had some reported success.

Over-the-counter medications—N-Acetyl cysteine 600 mg PO QD and vitamin C 500 mg PO QD. Also, do not forget Chantix in smokers, multivitamins with minerals, and CoQ10 or fish oil.

2. **Amphetamines**
Synthetic amphetamine derivatives have long been used to treat ADD, ADHD, and sleep disorders. When used orally, they have a slow onset of action but, effects can be longer-lasting. When given IV or smoked, it works very fast as it can quickly enter the brain. Ritalin and mephentermine (a banned performance-enhancing drug used by athletes) work similarly as they have a chemical structure close to methamphetamine. Because the brains of children and adolescents have not completed their development when these drugs are often prescribed legally, it remains to be seen if the use of these medications will have long-term effects in this population, which is a concern. In addition, there are many people in this age group who turn to either the many illegal chemical variations of these substances from easy to set

up Meth labs or use inordinate amounts of prescribed amphetamines to feed their abuse tendencies. Seizures can occur during methamphetamine use and withdrawal, so antiseizure treatment is necessary.

Most medications used for detoxification are similar to those available for cocaine dependence. The medications often used are as follows.

Methamphetamine substitution, the author uses slow-release methamphetamine (Concerta-54 mg/day), in decreasing/tapering doses if acceptable in your facility over a few weeks. Other amphetamine-derivative medications may be tried at the lowest effective dose and slowly tapered. In addition, Wellbutrin, Effexor (venlafaxine), and Cymbalta (duloxetine), which increase norepinephrine levels in the brain, have also been used as have short- or intermediate-acting benzodiazepines for anxiety and seizure control. Finally, modafinil has not, thus far, been shown to work well for amphetamine detoxification.

Naltrexone 50 mg PO, QD should be tried to aid in suppression of cravings.

Baclofen 20 mg TID can be helpful (the author uses 10 mg TID for the first 3 days, to minimize sedative effects). Baclofen may be used with naltrexone.

Keppra or Trileptal may be needed for seizure prevention/control and craving reduction.

3. Other stimulants: All should be treated in the same manner as above, using a combination of the same drugs, if medically necessary.

Amphetamine congeners—These drugs are exemplified by the medications used to treat ADD or ADHD.

Ephedrine/pseudoephedrine—A natural sympathomimetic amine, commonly used as a decongestant or short-term appetite suppressant. It is also used in the production of illegal methamphetamine.

Cathinones (bath salts)—A chemical derived from the leaf of an African shrub. They are chemically similar to ephedrine and amphetamine. Chewed in native form.

Yohimbine—From the bark of an African tree, this natural chemical has stimulant properties. It has been touted as an aphrodisiac or a sexual dysfunction treatment. Affects α-2 receptors. Increases amphetamine effects.

Caffeine—A mild CNS stimulatory agent capable of causing withdrawal. It is often abused in so-called "energy drinks" containing high concentrations of this stimulant. Most commonly abused by teenagers and young adults and has been associated with overdose and death. Consumption of these drinks correlates positively with tobacco usage.

Tobacco (nicotine)—A plant-derived stimulant that affects the α-4, β-2 receptors involved in the tolerance

and dependence on nicotine. Half-life is about 2 h, so withdrawal usually starts in the 2–3 h range. See smoking cessation withdrawal protocol presented later in this book (Section 4).

Bath salts—Cathinones (aminophenones) are amphetamine-like substances, which are synthetically derived from the plant *Catha edulis*, which grows on the Arab peninsula.

Flakka (α-PVP, sand)—A cathinone called $5 insanity, or poor persons cocaine because it is synthetic and cheap. Often comes from the Orient. Can be cut or mixed with other mainstream drugs. It contains α-PVP, a stimulant similar to other bath salts. Can be snorted, smoked, injected, or swallowed. Gives a euphoric "buzz," can cause high temperatures, paranoia, or acute and protracted psychosis. Without immediate attention, it can cause death, especially when mixed with other substances. It is said to be very toxic to kidneys, heart lungs, and brain.

Treatment can require intensive care unit admission.

Khat contains cathinone. It is derived from central African flowering plant.

MDMA (Ecstasy) and MDA are considered both stimulant and hallucinogen chemicals. MDA is a metabolite of MDMA. See hallucinogens below.

ADDICTION MANAGEMENT PROTOCOLS: BENZODIAZEPINES AND OTHER SEDATIVE-HYPNOTICS (DOWNERS)

Introduction

Benzodiazepines and other sedative-hypnotic medications impede CNS activity by initially affecting the inhibitory transmitter GABA pathway in the brain to increase its sedative action.

A single type of benzodiazepine, when used alone in prescribed doses, does not often cause serious medical consequences. However, when short-acting, quicker onset, high-potency ones are used IV (for enhanced euphoria) or in combination with other addictive substances (especially sedatives such as alcohol or opiate analgesics where they work in similar parts of the brain), an elevated mortality rate has been reported.

Relapses of withdrawal symptoms can often be seen months or even years after detoxification is completed, especially for patients with previous long-term, high-dose abuse.

Sedatives such as barbiturates are now less commonly used as they are being replaced by benzodiazepines, which are considered safer, are not associated with congenital malformations in pregnant women, and less prone to cause respiratory depression or abuse when properly used. However, as previously noted, they are still very dangerous if used in higher than prescribed doses or with other depressants.

Finally, methaqualone (Quaaludes, ludes, sopers), a synthetic barbiturate drug/depressant/sedative/muscle relaxant, which was popular in the 1960s and 1970s, which is now almost unheard of, is also capable of increasing GABA receptor activity and was the cause of side effects such as delirium, convulsions, hypertonia, kidney failure, and death by cardiac or respiratory arrest.

Intoxication by these medications has similar effects to alcohol overdose and can lead to seizures and delirium.

Treatment

The way the author usually classifies treatment of these medications is by length of use. In author's experience, use of these substances for less than 1 year often produced complete withdrawal within a shorter time frame, and use for more than 1 year was more likely to be associated with withdrawal lasting weeks or months after discontinuation. The taper for an overdose can necessitate inpatient therapy and the use of flumazenil, so short-term closer observation in a controlled environment may be necessary.

The use of a longer or slower taper, consisting of weeks (often 3−7) or months for withdrawal from this class of medications is usually required as follows.

It has been helpful in author's experience to try and substitute the same chemical, which the patient is abusing. (If the chemical is not known or mixed, it is usually started by using a fast-acting and more potent benzodiazepine [Ativan].) In addition, if patient has been on large doses of benzodiazepines, Ativan 1−2 mg can be used with caution as it seems to keep the patient more comfortable and less sick, and then switch to clonazepam 0.5−2 mg as the patient improves clinically. In those not using large doses of benzodiazepines, the taper is started with clonazepam in equivalent or close doses to what he/she has been using as it has a slower onset of action and less abuse potential. The dose is divided into 3−4 doses per day for those who have been using short-acting drugs and 1−3 doses per day for patients who have been using intermediate or longer-acting benzodiazepines.

The dose is decreased slowly to minimize side effects and often needs to go very slowly, by about 10% every 1−2 weeks. However, if the patient shows signs of drug toxicity-drooling, muscle in-coordination, slurred speech, etc., the medication is usually discontinued till the symptoms stop. The medication is then restarted at half the previous dose. After 50% of taper is completed, the taper usually needs to go even slower than before, often 10% every 2 weeks if signs of toxicity start to again appear at that time.

Propranolol 20 mg can be used PO TID-QID if symptoms of adrenergic signs of withdrawal occur and need suppression. Clonidine has not been found to be effective in the author's experience and is not recommended.

BuSpar (buspirone) 10 mg TID or 15 mg BID for anxiety. It is considered helpful because it is a nonbenzodiazepine anxiolytic medication and no cross-tolerance exists. However, it can take a while to work.

Keppra or Trileptal for seizure control should be initiated as seizures can occur during detoxification.

One of the previously mentioned sleep-promoting medications may be used if necessary (see previous opiate section).

Other drugs with potential use for detoxification:

1. Romazicon (flumazenil): A benzodiazepine receptor antagonist. It should be used in a controlled ER or inpatient setting. Its most important use is as a benzodiazepine rescue drug for those with benzodiazepine toxicity who are either losing consciousness or already unconscious. This medication is given IV in D5W or lactated Ringers solution at 0.1−0.2 mg for the first injection. Injections can be repeated at least four times if necessary. The reason why this medication is not routinely used for benzodiazepine detoxification is because it can cause precipitated withdrawal manifestations and trigger possible seizures.
2. Tegretol (carbamazepine): An antiseizure medication that has been used for alcohol and benzodiazepine detoxification. Dose is 200 mg TID for 7−10 days. It has a low abuse potential and few cognitive side effects.
3. Depakote (divalproex): May be as helpful in sedative-hypnotic withdrawal as it is for alcohol. Usual starting dose is 250 mg QD. Has many side effects. Use carefully with topiramate.

ADDICTION MANAGEMENT PROTOCOLS
Marijuana, Natural, and Synthetic Products
Introduction

Cannabis is a product of the hemp plant with about a 120-day growth cycle. The three most commonly used natural forms of this plant are marijuana, hashish, and hash oil. They contain many cannabinoids with the chemical tetrahydrocannabinol (THC) being the primary psychoactive component. (There are more than 500 psychoactive components in marijuana with 104 being cannabinoids.) Using genetic engineering, today's strains contain 30% THC or higher. Hashish is even more concentrated. It is usually smoked, vaped, or eaten (in candied form), and its major effect is cognitive impairment or "relaxation." Its effects can last up to 8 h due to inconsistent absorption and/or slow metabolism. Marijuana is the most commonly used illicit substance and has been associated with an increasing number of emergency room visits in recent years (especially motor vehicle accidents) and high consumption rates among college students. Thus far, there is no proven or FDA-recognized role for use of this substance (although it has been touted to help a number of medical conditions). Unfortunately, despite the lack of scientific evidence, marijuana is viewed by a majority of US adults as being beneficial in one way or another. It is now either completely legal or medically approved and available in many states.

Cannabinoid chemicals, mediated in the brain by the well-described, but poorly understood, endocannabinoid system, work in the frontal areas of the brain where they produce their addictive neuroadaptive changes by attaching to the cannabinoid receptor CB1, which they stimulate. The other receptor in this class CB2 is said to have a role in immune system modulation. The effects are somewhat similar to those of short-acting opiates. The cause of the "munchies" by cannabis is thought to be produced by an increase in the effect of an intestinal hormone, ghrelin (the hunger hormone), which is then able to act as a neurotransmitter within the brain. The neuroadaptive changes such as its negative effect on motivational behaviors, focus, or executive function have been known to occur for up to 24−48 h postfeelings of the "high." Chronic use may be associated with long-term cognitive or psychiatric problems. The jury is still out concerning the use of this chemical for chronic noncancer pain and its effects on the developing brain. However, the use of a non−THC cannabinoid formulation has recently gained FDA approval for certain types of childhood seizure control. Finally, recent reports indicate that marijuana use should be avoided in pregnancy and lactating women because of its potential harm to the fetus, which appears to be capable of profound deleterious effects on brain development, infant neurobehavior, and normal childhood CNS maturation.

Genetically engineered natural marijuana and synthetic marijuana (black mamba, K2, Spice, etc.) are also now being produced illegally.

Synthetic marijuana is a "designer" psychoactive substance chemically distinct from natural marijuana. It does not cross-react in the usual, natural marijuana chemical assay. Thus, it is designed to avoid urine detection, especially by law enforcement. The effects of genetically engineered and synthetic cannabinoids are said to mimic the effect of natural cannabinoids but are longer acting, more intense, and severe than the natural varieties of marijuana.

Side effects of synthetic marijuana include hypertension, possible myocardial infarction, agitation, seizures, and vomiting. Synthetic marijuana is capable of producing psychotic effects or intensification of other psychotic disorders.

Marijuana has also been deemed a "gateway substance" in addition to alcohol and nicotine. Recent research reports indicate that it may be capable of increasing the desire or enhance the vulnerability to try other substances, especially cigarettes due to being inhaled or by promoting chemical changes within the brain, especially in younger users. This is supported by the fact that the incidence of marijuana usage and other drug or alcohol disorders increases threefold and twofold for nicotine dependence. Finally, continuous use of marijuana has been associated with cognitive defects similar to ADHD and panic attacks, other psychiatric comorbidities. Little is known of its long-term effects. It is noted to be the most common substance associated with motor vehicle accidents.

Thus far, there has been little to no proven role for psychotherapeutic treatment after natural marijuana use but may be needed after synthetic marijuana overdose. Nevertheless, increasing numbers of research studies are finally being approved, funded, and conducted on both the short- and long-term side effects of marijuana (both the cannabinoid THC and the many others found in this plant) in the CNS, as the answers may have important clinical implications. In fact, it has already been reported that legalized marijuana or CBD oil (made from a cannabinoid with little or no THC) use may be useful in decreasing opioid prescribing rates. However, a lot of research needs to be done before this can become a reality.

Treatment

In the author's experience, it is rare to have to treat patients with detoxification medications admitted for marijuana use. The current medical literature does contain medications that have been shown to be helpful are as follows. These include (1) agonist therapies that mimic some effects of these drugs and are able to diminish cannabis consumption and attenuate the effects of withdrawal and cravings and (2) antagonist pharmacotherapies that block the CB1 receptor, so it cannot be stimulated by THC, has been shown to reduce withdrawal symptoms and decrease the choice to self-administer cannabis. These include the following:

1. Nabilone (Cesamet)—A long-acting, synthetic analogue of THC, is a potential prime agonist therapy. It is currently FDA approved for chemotherapy-induced nausea. It is still in development.
2. Naltrexone—An antagonist therapy used for treating other substance disorders, may well be helpful in increasing GABA biosynthesis, and may attenuate cannabis withdrawal by increasing GABA transmission, a major regulatory of brain system.
3. Gabapentin—1200 mg/day for 12 weeks. It is an antagonist therapy.
4. N-Acetylcholine—1200 mg BID for 8 weeks. It upregulates and restores glutamate activity disrupted by chronic drug use.
5. BuSpar—The nonbenzodiazepine antianxiety medication has been used in doses up to 60 mg/day for 12 weeks for cannabis withdrawal therapy.
6. In general, there is no proven place for either antidepressants or antipsychotics in cannabis treatment.
7. Smoking cessation therapy may also be used to curb the desire to smoke both nicotine and marijuana (see Section 4).

OTHER, EUPHORIA, RELAXATION SUBSTANCES

Kava—It is a product of the root of a plant from the western Pacific islands. Chewing this root leads to its sedative/anesthetic properties. It potentiates GABA but not DA or serotonin receptors. Its effects can last for hours to days. It is capable of producing liver toxicity. Treat, if necessary, like marijuana.

ADDICTION MANAGEMENT PROTOCOLS
Anabolic Steroids
Introduction
Anabolic steroids are now a schedule 111 controlled substances, which are only FDA approved for use in men who lack or have low testosterone levels in conjunction with an associated medical condition.

Nevertheless, they are frequently abused to try and enhance athletic performance or fitness and by body builders. It positively affects muscle and weight development. Steroid abuse is also associated with promotion of social rewards. Abusers can either use pharmacologic doses of natural testosterone and its derivatives or stronger synthetic varieties, clandestinely produced, to try and avoid detection. The use of large doses of either oral or injected anabolic steroids is associated with sexual side effects such as testicular or breast atrophy, decreased libido, in addition to gynecomastia, myocardial infarction, heart failure, stroke, hostility aggression, and hepatotoxicity. Other side effects include hypertension, insomnia, anorexia, psychosis, growth retardation in growing adolescents, and restlessness. Withdrawal effects such as depression, fatigue, and cravings are common. The FDA has just approved a class-wide labeling change for all testosterone products.

Treatment
The protocol for treating steroid abuse is first to stop the steroid being used. Because the chemical itself and the effects of anabolic steroids often last for months, one can substitute injectable doses of testosterone enanthate, 200 mg/ml, 1 mL every 2 weeks for 1 month and then slowly taper the dose to 1 cc each month for 2 months, and then 1/2 cc/month for 2 months. Short-term antipsychotic medications such as Thorazine, starting at 25−50 mg BID-TID and then slowly tapering the dose can be used for symptoms of mania or psychosis. In addition, short-term benzodiazepines can be used for panic or anxiety and then replaced by longer-term SSRI or SNRI therapy if needed for depression.

ADDICTION MANAGEMENT PROTOCOLS
Inhalants, Hallucinogens/Dissociatives
Introduction

1. Inhalants—These include chemicals that are breathable vapors, gases, aerosols, and solvents. They cause a form of a depressant, alcohol-like inebriated state in users, which includes hallucinations, euphoria, loss of consciousness, and respiratory depression. More commonly used are by young people who inhale the vapors from an inhalant-filled balloon. The author has also seen breathing cessation and death from hairspray inhalation. They both act and are expelled quickly through the lungs. Treatment includes removal of the offending inhalant and symptomatic therapy. Antipsychotics and benzodiazepines may be necessary.
2. Hallucinogens/dissociatives—Often loosely referred to as club or designer drugs. They are a large and growing group of synthetic substitutes of other often abused substances. They commonly bind to the serotonin receptor. Their actions within the CNS include dissociation between mind and body, hallucinations (usually visual), memory defects/amnesia, and thought/mind alterations. They are capable of neurotoxicity and have a high abuse potential. Effects often last 3−6 h. Included within this

group are PCP, dextromethorphan (DMX, triple Cs)—a synthetic opiate derivative with antitussive effects (but minimal opiate ones), which can be purchased over the counter and have PCP-like effects in large doses, MDMA (Ecstasy), MDA, ketamine (an old anesthetic medication and "rave drug," which is currently being reinvestigated as a rapid-acting antidepressant, N-methyl D—aspartame receptor antagonist, mescaline, psilocybin (magic mushrooms), another hallucinogen, euphoric being investigated for its potential antidepression, anxiety effects, ibogaine, an illegal US schedule 1 drug, used in other countries as a possible opiate addiction treatment, GHB (γ-hydroxy butyrate, a precursor and metabolite of GABA), flunitrazepam (Rohypnol, Roofies, date rape drug)—an intermediate-acting benzodiazepine lasting 4—6 h and can cause amnesia and LSD. They are often not detected in standard urine presumptive toxicology screens and thus can present difficult diagnostic problems. However, current investigation indicates a potential helpful role for treating mental health disorders. An example of this is the ongoing evaluation of low-dose MDMA for treating PTSD.

Treatment

Treatment is symptomatic with supportive care and sometimes the need for fast-acting benzodiazepines (although longer-acting benzodiazepines have been used successfully for the longer-acting substances such as GHB) or ventilation therapy.

Special Populations

In the author's opinion, four specific groups of people warrant special emphasis and attention as their needs and specific challenges presented often differ from most of the patients who need help with their substance abuse disorders. These populations include pregnant women, the criminal justice system, adolescents, and military personnel.

Substance Abuse in Pregnancy

Substance abuse during a pregnancy, which is now occurring with increasing frequency in our adolescent and adult population, even if only involving tobacco use, should be considered a high-risk event.

The problems that the administration of abusable substances can present to the mother and developing fetus include the production of a multitude of well-described adverse and often severe gestational consequences such as hypoxia and fetal distress.

In addition, they appear to be responsible for causing a number of well-defined sequelae, immediately

postpartum as exemplified by neonatal withdrawal syndrome due to maternal substance use.

Finally, according to the medical literature, increasing rates of pregnant women with opioid use disorder in the hospital for delivery, foster care placement, future childhood learning impediments, psychiatric issues, and even the possibility of an increased propensity for eventual adolescent or adult substance abuse from gestational brain impairment have been documented.

Substance use may occur in a single pregnancy, but multiple pregnancy addictions are well recognized. The abused substances involved include one or more of the spectrum of natural or synthetic chemicals previously mentioned within this section, from opiates and alcohol to benzodiazepines, stimulants, psychedelics, and even nicotine.

As a general rule, most substances of abuse can be withdrawn during pregnancy under the guidance of the addiction team. The major exception is opiates where affected individuals are placed on methadone or buprenorphine (preferably) throughout gestation. Medications used to reduce or eliminate substance abuse cravings are either contraindicated or have not been properly tested and approved for use in pregnant women with the exception of a recent report that indicates that even higher doses of buprenorphine do not increase neonatal abstinence syndrome (NAS) severity.

Although self-motivation to discontinue the use of the addicting substance(s), which has been known to occur after the pregnancy has been recognized, it often takes appropriate referral and the support of a specialized, experienced addiction team, residential lodging, and hospital, all ideally within close proximity to each other.

The members of this team should include not only a specialized addiction medicine physician and licensed, experienced, healthcare professionals but also a host of other medical specialists including an obstetrician/gynecologist with advanced training in perinatology, whose practice focuses on the care of high-risk pregnant women. In addition, neonatologists with newborn addiction treatment experience and an appropriate Newborn Intensive Care Unit for treatment of neonatal abstinence syndrome (NAS), which usually develops in newborns within 2—3 days of birth due to in utero exposure to opioids, are an important part of the treatment progression of addicted, pregnant women. Units capable of handling neonatal withdrawal and other possible congenital or other reported complications of substance abuse are absolutely invaluable.

Further supplementary nonphysician medical professionals are also needed to ensure that proper complete care is given to the pregnant mother, so her multiple special needs can be met, predelivery, and for aftercare of both the mother and baby post delivery.

The availability of proximate lodging during pregnancy and maternal and infant care after gestation may also constitute a major concern because a healthy pregnancy outcome is best ensured with easily obtained, regular, pre- and postdelivery medical attention, substance abuse counseling, wholesome meal planning, proper exercise, vitamin and medication use, plus protective and compassionate individualized personal care.

Often, without proper private insurance coverage or adequate personal financial resources to obtain this type of care, this goal has been very difficult to accomplish.

In addition, depending on the substance used, the possibility of breastfeeding may also need to be addressed by a qualified health professional at the appropriate time within the entire process.

Lastly, the use of pharmacotherapy, if needed for only a short period of time or during the entire pregnancy (depending on the type and amount of the primary substance used), requires careful consideration and monitoring, as many medications currently used for substance abuse treatment or detoxification are contraindicated in pregnant women.

Theoretically, other helpful medications may be considered, but their safety and efficacy have been poorly studied to date in pregnancy or, due to FDA regulation, must be employed with special caution during gestation.

Finally, patient legal issues may also be a complicating factor and must be taken into consideration by the treatment team.

The Criminal Justice System

In general, our current criminal justice system appears quite antiquated when dealing with the substance abuse population, which, in the author's opinion, is severely complicating our ability to assist with both short- and long-term substance abuse epidemic intervention and treatment in this population.

Owing to this lack of understanding and its traditionally tough and punitive approach to substance abusers and their comorbidities, this system has become overtaxed at all levels including arrest, court, trial, and incarceration being all too common despite available innovative improvements in ways of approaching and intervening early in this problem. As exemplified by the power of social service agencies, they often, but sadly, have the ability to remove children of thoroughly capable parents who are using and doing well on treatment medications as part of their redemption program.

This archaic disciplinary system too often fails to properly discriminate between hardened criminals who need to be separated from society and those individuals who are in possession of only minimal amounts of substance and certainly nonviolent, who merit rehabilitation efforts.

In addition, arrest or criminal records can "follow" a person, although rehabilitated, and act as a disqualifying or hindering factor, for the duration of their rebuilt life.

Those incarcerated must tolerate extreme, painful withdrawal, which can by itself be fatal. Those who relapse after release from jail, due to a diminution of tolerance, are at least 10 times more likely to have a fatal overdose because the system often fails to provide effective assisted medication treatment or addiction therapy services before, while incarcerated or after release. The result is that they again will likely return to a life of addiction and crime which the chance of treatment may avert. This problem is finally being slowly addressed in some criminal justice systems as abbreviated below.

This program, incorporating a collaborative, nonjudgmental, treatment referral-oriented approach, between the community and the criminal justice system, called Drug Treatment Court (DTC) to therapeutically help substance abusers before, in, and after incarceration, has recently been developed and appears effective, although still far from universally available. This program encompasses many of the traditional medication management and mental health therapy approaches commonly found in programs outside the criminal justice system.

In conclusion, additional substance abuse understanding, education, and treatment should be funded, incorporated, and mandatory for those professionals involved at all levels of the criminal justice system, plus the incorporation of innovative DTC type and other rehabilitative methods for substance abuse to those currently affected. These methods should then be integrated into the new updated and innovative intervention strategies with a focus on self-reliance and rehabilitation being the ultimate goal of the process for affected individuals.

Adolescent Substance Abuse and Treatment

Adolescence is an intense and trying time period during the life of an individual.

Throughout the duration of adolescence, there is increased somatic and CNS growth and developmental progression. The brain undergoes many anatomic and chemical alterations till its development is completed sometime in the early adult age range.

These modulations include, but are not limited to, behavioral maturation, parental separation, attaining autonomy and independence, image adjustment, personal identity, and even rebellion against authority.

Typically, substance experimentation begins in the early to midportion of adolescent development, most commonly due to normal increased adolescent "risky" or adventuresome behaviors by recreational means among friends and other social contacts.

In vulnerable individuals, due to a combination of genetic and/or environmental factors, substance use is becoming a growing public health problem, as it increases in prevalence, proceeding from that point earlier in adolescence to intensified use and/or true abuse/addiction in later adolescent or adult life.

Cooccurring, but unrecognized or treated, mental health problems appear to be implicated in the development of further enhancement of the reward circuitry by promoting additional dopamine production.

Adolescents often first start with clandestine access to substances such as alcohol or cigarette smoking and then go on to experimenting with marijuana (which is why they are called the gateway drugs) before moving on to other addictive substances, which may also involve nonmedical prescription diversion or certain pleasure-deriving OTC medications.

A comprehensive individualized assessment will usually provide the basis for determination of the severity of the substance abuse problem, the need for possible treatment and the level of treatment necessary.

Informed consent, parental consent, and confidentiality are areas of treatment important to address between the physician, healthcare professionals, state law, and patient. These relationships are often complicated and even confounded by individual state laws, which may regulate, dictate, and control the role played and decisions made by the patient; healthcare providers; and parents, guardians, or custodians during the assessment and treatment process, especially in case of patient incompetence.

Pharmacologic treatment and mental health counseling are generally similar to that of an adult but must be individualized based on patient maturity and understanding.

Military Personnel and Veterans

With firsthand knowledge, the author is well aware of the serious problems faced by the active US military, national guard, veterans, and military families/dependants, especially concerning alcohol plus other misused or abused substances (which have actually been a problem for centuries but has recently escalated in extent). In fact, recent government reports note that the rate of substance abuse, especially alcohol consumption and binge drinking in this population, is double that of the general population and veterans are twice as likely as nonveterans to die from accidental overdoses of highly addictive painkillers due to chronic pain.

The military, to correctly perform its mission, must always be in a heightened state of readiness. However, staying at this necessarily intensified level of alertness is continuously being impacted by the physical and emotional stresses placed on those in uniform due to deployments, combat situations, and ongoing changes in duty stations and assignments, which are responsible for long periods of time when these soldiers must be away from critical support systems necessary to maintain peak physical and emotional health.

Thus, besides the previously mentioned internal pressures, pain from injury or battle, and tension faced by soldiers on active duty and later as veterans, cooccurring issues of stress within their families appear to also play a role in the probability of developing a substance use problem (and potentially also PTSD) in any member of both the close and remote segments of the complete military household unit. Unfortunately, PTSD has been linked to heart disease, which is the leading cause of death in veterans. Therefore, simultaneous substance abuse and PTSD treatment is especially important in the military and veteran community.

Furthermore, any coexistent but undiscovered mental disorder, with or without the occurrence of physical injury or pain, in a person on active duty or after discharge, can add substantially to the onset of a problem of alcohol or substance abuse, prevention, screening, or efforts at successful rehabilitation.

Finally, another confounding issue thwarting the rehabilitation process in active duty military personnel has been the previous, and even continued, treatment of substance abuse as a disciplinary offense rather than understanding that it is a treatable chronic brain disorder, which deserves medical and therapeutic attention rather than reprimand.

At this time, each branch of the military and the VA have systems in place to intercede before, during, and after this type of problem may occur in a service member or a close family member. Nevertheless, these organizations lack adequate personnel and monetary support/resources, at this time, to better help all of those in need at each step of the complete rehabilitation process.

It is hoped that the President and Congress will do more than give mostly "lip service" to this serious problem by appropriating all the funds necessary to help those who have given so much for their country to be able to overcome this service connected, debilitating disorder and regain their proper place in society.

Addiction Management Protocols: Smoking Cessation Management

Nicotine Replacement and Prescription Medication

BACKGROUND

In 2000, there were an estimated 4.1 million premature deaths in the world attributed to tobacco use (and the leading cause of death in the United States), which includes smoking, chewing tobacco, snuff, or other finely chopped or smokeless tobacco, all of which have equal addictive properties. In fact, in 2015, despite the rapidly growing death rate from opiates, tobacco was responsible for approximately 15 times that number. This equates to 5 million years of potential life lost that year. The most unfortunate facts these statistics convey are not only that the deaths of so many of these people occurred during the most population-based productive years of their lives but also that these deaths were preventable and unnecessary.

In the United States, cigarette smoking is responsible for 25% of all deaths. However, although overall smoking rates have declined, about 20% of US adults still smoke, and 22% of adolescents in the 12th grade are affected by this expectant future disabling condition. In addition, smoking has been reported in 74% of people, 12 years and older who received recent SUD treatment, three times higher than people who did not receive treatment during the same period of time, and people with mental and substance abuse disorders are approximately twice as likely to smoke cigarettes and/or vape than the rest of the general population. Thus, they are more likely to die from smoking-related illness than mental or substance use disorders. Finally, although difficult and specially challenging in the substance abuse population, smoking cessation in the author's experience can be accomplished successfully, leading to a reduced risk of smoking-related diseases and improvement in behavioral health outcomes.

For those addicted to this substance, nicotine appears to work in the central nervous system by attaching to α-2, β-2 receptors and then altering the levels of certain brain neurotransmitters to calm, produce stress relief, and soothe those hooked to sustain the addiction/dependence and suppress or prevent withdrawal symptoms. Finally, nicotine is classified as a legal, reinforcement-enhancing type of substance because once a cigarette is smoked, withdrawal will occur sometime in the near future, usually about 2 h. This then induces that person to smoke another cigarette to relieve the unpleasant upcoming withdrawal symptoms and reinforce the pleasurable feeling generated within the brain from a fresh infusion of the substance. An understanding of this concept becomes especially important in those who are undergoing detoxification for other addicting substance because the object of helping the patient prevent relapse is made much more difficult when a legal reinforcing drug continues to be used during and after the detoxification process for other abused substances, because it still facilitates a continuous/repetitive behavior, which supports the potential resumption of previous illegal drug consumption.

SOME ADDITIONAL IMPORTANT FACTS

1. Three-quarters of the deaths from smoking are in men, but the death rate in women is rising.
2. Many smokers use and continue to use tobacco products, in part, for weight loss and weight control, especially overweight smokers.
3. Smoking is highly addictive—actually more than marijuana. In fact, addiction has been reported to occur before a person smokes a full pack of 20 cigarettes. In addition, 95% of adult smokers began smoking before they reached 21 years of age.
4. Smokers usually die 5—15 years earlier than never-smokers.
5. Smokers live to enjoy all the pleasure that nicotine can afford (stimulation and relaxation) but die from the tar in cigarettes that slowly destroys their lungs.

6. Nicotine affects all organs of the body. Smokers have twice the risk of fatal heart disease, 10 times the risk of lung cancer, and several times the risk of other cancers, which have now been tied directly to their cigarette addiction.

7. Smokers have higher rates of stroke, an increased osteoporosis risk, bone fractures, dementia, lung disease, erectile dysfunction, alcohol abuse, yellow-stained fingers, and typically develop severely wrinkled skin at a young age. Smoking accounts for the primary cause of house fire mortality.

8. About 90% of COPD, a type of severe, chronic lung disease, causing an inability to breathe properly, occurs in smokers. A recent scientific study reveals that the faster the daily nicotine content is reduced, the faster the biomarkers of smoke exposure on the body organs decrease, which translates into longer and healthier lives for this patient population.

9. The children of smokers often have lower birth weights and increased perinatal and neonatal mortality, are more likely to be mentally retarded, and have more frequent respiratory problems and lung infections, in addition to an increased incidence of ear infections.

10. In the author's opinion, a recent excellent publication by Substance Abuse and Mental Health Services Administration (SAMSHA) clearly details the reason to combine smoking cessation and substance abuse treatment as it increases the odds of long-term recovery, may have mental health benefits, the physical health benefits begin almost immediately, and helps SUD patients better focus on a positive lifestyle.

11. Smokers who quit by age 35 add an additional number of years to their life span, and even older smokers can benefit in this regard, as the risk of death starts decreasing shortly after cessation of this substance.

12. Tobacco is infused with thousands of chemicals, mostly additives of which about 100 are very toxic or carcinogenic.

13. Smoking causes its detrimental effects on the human body in three ways: (1) primary smoking problems that often detrimentally affects one or multiple organs in the smokers themselves; (2) secondary smoke that causes problems in the people who inhale the smoke by continuously being in close contact with the smokers themselves, especially family members including children. Furthermore, second-hand smoke has also been reported to be capable of initiating nicotine addiction in those affected, and (3) tertiary problems caused by the residue or particles of burning cigarettes or smoking itself that can recirculate into the air after first landing on the skin, hair, and clothing of smokers in addition to other objects in the environment. It can then be inhaled by someone who comes into contact with these again floating airborne particles with the potential of causing detrimental effects on them.

14. Smoking addiction remains one of the world's most challenging public health problems and is extremely undertreated.

15. The FDA is considering lowering the nicotine content in cigarettes to nonaddictive levels.

MEDICAL TREATMENT OF SMOKING ADDICTION
Introduction
Pharmacologic therapy to aid in smoking cessation (again linked with counseling), as recently published by the National Comprehensive Cancer Network, is effective as it has been shown to at least double the chance of successfully quitting. All forms of medical substitution therapy reduce the amount of nicotine at brain nicotine receptors and have about the same level of success. Higher rates of success can be achieved with combination of more than one form of substitution therapy and with the prescription medications Zyban and especially Chantix, which also work at the brain nicotine receptor level (and actually may help with all addictive substance detoxification as they act at the same area of the brain) to control the desire to smoke. The prescription medications Zyban and Chantix contain no nicotine. Often, those motivated to quit smoking will experience weight gain because nicotine promotes weight loss. As discussed above, methods for smoking cessation include substitution therapy (nicotine patches, gum, and lozenges), which are available over the counter; e-cigarettes, which are available at stores and on the Internet; and prescription medications, which include bupropion (Zyban) and varenicline (Chantix). The success of each of these agents appears to work by boosting brain dopamine and norepinephrine levels and thus mimicking the effects of nicotine.

These agents should only be offered to those smokers who have been identified as motivated to quit smoking and are ready to do so.

Other warnings include patients with heart problems or high blood pressure, as nicotine can increase heart rate; stomach ulcer; diabetes; or those on a salt-restricted diet. Medical contraindications include women who are pregnant or breastfeeding, in addition to adolescents. These agents should also be kept away from children and pets. Patients should also plan for and take measures to prevent the anticipated weight gain. The commonly available methods for smoking cessation are as follows.

Substitution Therapy

1. The nicotine patch is quite appropriate as a form of primary therapy for smoking cessation in those with normal hearts (no irregular beats, recent heart problems, or medication-controlled high blood pressure). The patch is generally applied each 24 h for approximately 12 weeks or less but can be used for longer periods. The patches are usually dosed according to the number of cigarettes smoked daily and degree of addiction. Adults smoking more than 15 cigarettes per day usually start using 21 mg (or 24 mg if available) patches. As noted above, usually one patch per day is needed, but occasionally two may be required (one patch per 12 hours). The patch strength is slowly decreased or tapered to 14 mg after 2–6 weeks and then 7 mg at 4–8 weeks. Patients who usually smoke no more than 15 cigarettes per day will generally start at a lower-dose nicotine patch (14 mg). Patches should be applied to dry, nonhairy skin. It should be noted that skin reactions from the patch have been reported in up to 50% of patients but are usually mild or self-limiting. The treatment for those skin reactions is cortisone cream. In patients with very sensitive skin, the patch may need to be discontinued. Please be aware that if you have vivid dreams or sleep disturbances, the patch should be removed at bedtime. Please watch for symptoms of nicotine overdose, which is described in the nicotine gum section. Generally, the patch is discontinued after 10 weeks. Each patch should not be worn for more than 24 h and never cut into half. After use, the patch should be taken off, sticky ends folded, and then discarded.

2. Nicotine gum is also used as primary therapy for smoking cessation over the same time frame as the patch. Again, the same precautions should be used with this form of therapy. Nicotine gum is available in doses of 2 and 4 mg. Patients who smoke 25 cigarettes per day or less and start smoking at least 30 min after waking up should generally start with a lower dose. Usually, the 4-mg-strength gum is reserved for patients who either smoke more than 25 cigarettes per day or have failed the 2 mg strength but remain motivated to quit. Do not eat or drink for 15 min before starting the gum or while chewing. The gum should be chewed until it causes a tingling sensation and then placed between the jaw and gum. Begin chewing again when the tingling stops, and repeat this process until the tingling feeling is almost gone. Repeat with the next piece of gum when cravings recur. Patients using the 2-mg-strength gum should not exceed 30 pieces per day, and those using the 4 mg strength should not exceed 20 pieces per day. Patients taking medication for depression or asthma need to be watched more closely as these problems can intensify. Please consult your physician if you develop mouth, tooth, or jaw problems; an irregular heartbeat; palpitations; nausea; dizziness; diarrhea; or weakness as they may indicate a nicotine overdose. Do not use the gum for longer than 12 weeks.

3. Nicotine lozenges are customarily used in the same way and have the same side effects as the patch and gum. They come in 2 and 4 mg strengths. After discarding the paper wrapper, the 2-mg-strength lozenge is most often used when a person's first cigarette is consumed after 30 min of waking up. The 4 mg lozenge is most often used if a person's first cigarette is smoked within 30 min of waking up. The lozenges are generally used every 1–2 h at first, and the dose is slowly decreased as dictated by treatment success (using them every 2–4 h and then every 4–8 h over an 8–9 or more weeks). The same at-risk populations as noted above should avoid use of this form of nicotine cessation therapy. The lozenges are usually consumed for a 10- to 12-week period.

Clinical Pearl

A recent study has indicated that using a patch combined with another type of substitution therapy (gum, lozenge) may be as effective as a prescription medication. One might wish to try this before considering a prescription form of smoking cessation.

4. E-cigarettes, often referred to as e-cigs, e-hookahs, mods, vape pens, vapes, JUULS, tank systems, etc., which have been gaining popularity as a diversified product group category, especially in teenagers, are a form of a battery-operated, atomized (an electronic device to vaporize nicotine) alternative to other forms of therapy as they merely deliver a heated, water-based aerosol vapor that contains flavoring, nicotine, or other additives. In 2017, about 50% more high school and middle school students vape rather than smoke. Additionally, "dripping," where the chemical is dropped directly onto the coil, has also become popular as it produces thicker clouds of vapor (a higher concentration of vaporized nicotine). E-cigarettes are most often used by young adults, 18–24 years of age. Their advantage stems

from the facts that they are cheaper, have the ability for the smoker to alter the voltage and heat, come in nicotine-free form, or can use real nicotine cartridges, in addition to various flavors, and lack most second- and third-hand smoke—induced long-term nicotine problems due to their decreased amount of tobacco residue, which makes the e-cigarette vapor less hazardous. However, a recent study has indicated that multiple carcinogenic chemicals have been found in the urine of e-cigarette smokers (and obviously would also appear in the vapor), which challenges this assumption.

5. In addition, the theory has been advanced that starting to use these devices at a young age may predispose an individual to lifelong nicotine or marijuana use rather than promotion of smoking cessation and cause decreased successful smoking cessation in adults who start vaping to accomplish this end.

Nicotine cartridges most commonly hold the same amount of nicotine as 1.5—2 packs of cigarettes. Some people like the fact that they appear to have "smoke" coming out of the end of the cigarette. The cartridge is usually discarded after the nicotine is used up and another is started. The problem with these cigarettes is due to the unknown types and amounts of chemicals in the device itself and its ingredients.

Although many of them were originally manufactured in the Orient, most are now manufactured and marketed by traditional tobacco companies. Additionally, a naturally occurring, nonpsychoactive component of cannabinoids (cannabidiol—CBD) oil has recently become available for use in e-cigarettes. It is said to be nondetectable in drug tests and advertised as an anxiety-relieving substance. However, it has been reported that it may also increase their desire to use or become addicted to these substances.

JUUL, another form of e-cigarette, is a slim black vaporizer which looks like a flash drive for a computer. It contains a small cartridge, called a pod, filled with multiple flavors of "juice" plus about the same amount of nicotine as a pack of cigarettes and a heating element, which vaporizes but does not burn tobacco. Thus, like a vape, it leaves no ashes. What it does is to dispense nicotine to a user in a supposedly healthier manner, without the hazardous tar and other foul-tasting cigarette ingredients.

Since 2016, the FDA has been regulating e-cigarettes as a tobacco product (without being subject to cigarette taxes), and e-cigarette companies have to submit a premarket tobacco application until 2022 to keep their products on the market. Furthermore, the FDA, recently, in response to the epidemically exploding number of youth, aged 12—17 using or open to using e-cigarettes, has initiated a major prevention campaign to protect America's youth from the dangers of using any tobacco or nicotine-containing products in addition to illegal sales of these products.

Finally, there is no regulation of nicotine or other chemical content (flavorings) or knowledge of what other harmful chemicals may be contained in these items. Thus, batches of the same product have been found to have highly variable levels of the nicotine delivered. They have been declared a health hazard by the US Surgeon General. Although a recent report indicates that e-cigarettes may indeed have the potential to help patients refrain from conventional cigarette smoking or quit smoking without side effects for up to 2 years, most experts still disagree and discourage its use because they have other data suggesting that these products can actually encourage subsequent tobacco use in youth, possibly due to its appealing flavors, and there are only limited data concerning the long-term safety, behavioral effects, or success in cessation studies available to date. This is supported by the recent demonstration of the nicotine concentration in e-liquid samples of the five most popular flavors, which found that there was clear and inaccurate nicotine concentration labeling in these solutions, which may pose a significant risk to consumers. Additionally, there is a significant and growing market for totally unregulated "look-alike products," which could contain hazardous materials. Thus, this method of smoking cessation remains unproven as a complete cessation tool, appears to be detrimental to a developing fetus, and may actually foster progression by young users to conventional tobacco products or other substances. In addition, it appears that about 75% of flavored cigarettes contain the potentially deadly chemical diacetyl, which is known to cause scarring of the air sacs leading to cough and shortness of breath or even death. Finally, e-cigarettes are a respiratory tract irritant, and there is a case report of an 18-month-old child who died from drinking a small amount of highly concentrated "e-juice."

6. A nasal spray product is also available for smoking cessation. It is only available by prescription. This product is beyond the scope of this book.

FDA-Approved Prescription Medications for Smoking Cessation

1. Bupropion SR (Zyban)

    Zyban is a form of the prescription, antidepressant medication bupropion (Wellbutrin SR) and an antagonist of the nicotine receptor. It has been successfully used for smoking cessation and proven effective. One must note that bupropion has also been used in diet medications as obesity appears to be controlled in the same areas of the brain that is responsible for addictive behaviors. The same cautions are present for this prescription drug with a special contraindication for individuals with a seizure disorder, pregnancy, history of an eating disorder, or active alcohol consumption, and those who are using another formulation of bupropion or who have used an MAO-inhibiting drug in the past 14 days as they inhibit dopamine (please check with your physician to see if you are currently taking one). It can also cause psychiatric symptoms. The usual dosage is 150 mg every morning for 3 days, then increasing to 150 mg twice per day (higher doses may promote seizures) for 7−24 weeks following the quit date. The drug is then stopped. Patients should use this medication for 1−2 weeks before they quit smoking. The most common side effects using this medication are insomnia (sleeping difficulties), gastrointestinal problems, and dry mouth. Sometimes Zyban has been used in combination with a nicotine patch, but this combination can produce nicotine withdrawal symptoms (depression, agitation) and is therefore not recommended.

2. Varenicline (Chantix)

    Chantix tablets are a prescription medication that is considered the most effective for smoking cessation (and also may be effective for all abused substances). Chantix works by binding to the nicotine receptor to control cravings (it is a partial stimulant of the nicotine receptor and therefore blocks nicotine from activating the receptor—not allowing nicotine to bind to the receptor). Chantix also stimulates the dopamine reward system, so the need to smoke is diminished. It is usually started 1 week before the cigarette quit date. The patient starts by using one 0.5-mg tablet each morning for the first 3 days. If tolerated well, 0.5-mg tablets are then used twice per day for the next 4 days. The medication is administered after eating, with a glass of water. On day 7, begin 1 mg of the drug twice per day for a total of 12 weeks. A second course of this drug has also been used in special circumstances. Chantix should then be stopped. Generally, the most common side effects of this drug are similar to those of Zyban and usually gastrointestinal in nature. Chantix has some other occasional/infrequent potential serious side effects such as severe depression and suicidal thoughts and acts, recurrence of preexisting psychosis, as well as agitation, anxiety psychosis, strange dreams, paranoia, hallucinations, hostility, and homicidal thoughts. In addition, sudden heart issues have been reported. If any of these occur, the medication should be stopped immediately and reported to your physician. Finally, alcohol is thought to intensify Chantix side effects. The FDA has recently released a warning that Chantix can change the way people react to alcohol due to its interaction with this substance. Thus, patients taking this medication *must* greatly decrease or hopefully eliminate their alcohol consumption. In addition, the FDA warning reemphasized the rare seizures caused by this medication and its neuropsychiatric side effects on mood, behavior, and thinking ability. It is not generally recommended to start in conjunction with substitution therapy.

3. Nortriptyline (Sensoval, Aventyl, Pamelor, Norpress, Allegron, Noritren, Nortrilen), another prescription medication, has also been used as a smoking cessation agent, but it is not FDA approved for this application.

4. Clonidine—small studies noted a favorable response to this prescription medication for smoking cessation.

Clinical Pearl

If one or more substitution type of medications fail to work, try Chantix first, and possibly with a combination of a substitution product as improved results have been reported, but watch the patient closely for side effects.

Addiction Management Protocols: Long-Term Medication Abstinence Options to Help Curb Substance Abuse Relapse

INTRODUCTION

Although complete abstinence is always the goal of substance abuse treatment, cravings are part of the substance addiction-withdrawal-relapse process. They are caused by the previously produced abnormal changes in the brain, which are responsible for executive functioning. These changes, which can clearly occur from substance abuse, are capable of short-circuiting normal brain patterns, so abusers will continue to have the urge to again start using substances (relapse). Cravings can be caused by many things including depression, anxiety, memories of previous exposure, or environmental anticipatory drug cues/reminders, such as past "people, places, and things," which are capable of triggering the urge to use, especially in the first 6 months after total substance detoxification. Avoidance of these biologic or environmental stimuli, in addition to continued psychotherapy and the use of anticraving medications, is considered the primary key to success and the beginning of a substance-free life after detoxification and withdrawal.

Cravings can be extremely intense, and that is why programs such as MAT have been successful to date. Although many medications have been reported to help curb cravings from addictive substances, there are now a growing number of commonly used medications available, which have been the most extensively tested and shown to successfully help, circumvent, or prevent the onset of cravings in susceptible individuals for at least a single substance, and often more. These underprescribed and underused medications appear to act in those areas of the brain known to help improve decision-making and assist those vulnerable to withstand the temptation(s) to use. It is recommended by the NIH that medications for alcohol treatment should be discontinued if alcohol continues to be consumed 4–6 weeks after treatment initiation. Baclofen, gabapentin, and ondansetron appear to be the best options for patients with liver disease.

OFTEN ASKED QUESTIONS

Before considering any of these medications, a few things should be clarified:

1. Do these medications work? You bet they can. However, you must remember that no medication works for everyone. In addition, most relapse appears to occur if these medications are stopped or discontinued and long-term psychotherapy is not maintained. Furthermore, many of the currently approved medications are more than 10 years old. New, potentially helpful craving prevention medications are currently in development but unfortunately, while potentially promising, are not yet proven for this application. That is why each person needs to find the one(s) that work best for their cravings and continue taking these particular medication(s). It must also be remembered that many of these medications are not substitutes for the substance but influence the desire to use them, by moderating their effects or stopping their use by curbing cravings.

2. Have each of these medications been tested to see if they work on all abused substances? No, but most of them appear to have the potential to do so because they may help reestablish normalized frontal lobe and limbic system brain chemistry. Naltrexone, disulfiram, and acamprosate are considered first-line medications (FDA approved—especially for alcohol) because of the volume of scientific evidence available, whereas others are thought of as second-line treatment options when naltrexone or acamprosate is not found to be effective.

Addiction Medicine for Health Care Professionals. https://doi.org/10.1016/B978-0-323-68017-2.00005-3

3. Can these medications cause serious side effects? Yes, although not very common, they can occur. Thus, it is important to remember that your doctor is only prescribing these medications because he/she believes that the benefits outweigh their potential side effect risk. In addition, if any of the serious side effects appear (mental/mood changes/clinical symptoms such as depression or suicidal thoughts, possible kidney problems, fainting, rapid heartbeat, nonstopping diarrhea, vision or hearing changes), please report them to your doctor immediately. Finally, your doctor may require you to take periodic laboratory tests while you are using one or more of these medications to see if any organs are being adversely affected.

4. Do these medications begin to work immediately? It should be noted that these medications may take a few days to weeks to work properly and may cause temporary side effects such as drowsiness or gastro-intestinal problems. As noted above, the medical literature indicates that relapses most often occur if and when the medication is stopped. These medications may also need to be initiated on less than a complete dose to minimize temporary side effects.

5. Should antidepressants and benzodiazepines be used for patients with an alcohol use disorder? The American Psychiatric Association guidelines recommend *against* the use of these medications, except for situations where a cooccurring disorder requires treatment in a facility where their interaction can be carefully monitored and appropriately adjusted.

6. Are these long-term relapse prevention medications supported by the insurance companies? Absolutely, because the insurers would rather pay for one of these medications than for more expensive in- and/or outpatient treatment after a relapse.

7. What potential relapse prevention medications are under development? These fit into a number of categories. Potential vaccines or other medications to prevent or ameliorate drug addiction are currently under development. Their purpose is to diminish reinforcement by methods such as blocking blood−brain barrier crossing of addictive substances or prevent attachment of the substance to the receptor.

8. Are scheduled physician and therapist visits important? As indicated above, they are the cornerstones of successful long-term sobriety maintenance. Please be sure to keep all scheduled doctor's appointments while using these medications in addition to attending your regular counseling and support group sessions.

9. Should emergency naloxone (Narcan) be available to all opiate patients currently in recovery? It is extremely important that all patients who complete either a total detoxification or MAT program be discharged with a take-home opioid overdose kit. This medication should always be kept either on their person or in close proximity for immediate use, and family, friends, and companions should also be educated in its application.

FDA APPROVED LONG-TERM ANTI-CRAVING MEDICATION
Naltrexone (Revia, Vivitrol)
This medication is a cousin of the drug naloxone (Narcan), an opiate blocker (nonselective antagonist of mu, kappa, and delta receptors), which is used to treat patients who overdose on opiates by blocking opioid receptors and moderating the dopamine effects for opiates and the endorphin-mediated reward effects for alcohol. It is FDA approved. It can alleviate/reduce cravings and the pleasurable effects of opiates and alcohol (in addition to others) and therefore reduce their use, especially heavy drinking. It must be remembered, however, that if someone stops the medication and has a relapse, serious consequences such as respiratory arrest or even death can occur due to loss of previous tolerance. Naltrexone use is contraindicated in patients with liver failure or severe hepatitis (especially if higher doses are contemplated). Therefore, check liver chemistries before using. It is one of the most clinically tested of all the anticraving medications; it is considered a first-line medication by the American Psychiatric Association for an opiate and alcohol use disorder, and that is why the author usually uses this medication first. It comes in two forms, a pill (ReVia) and an injection (Vivitrol). The pill generally lasts for 24 h, and the effects of the injection will persist for 1 month. Naltrexone should *only* be started after all opiates have been cleared from the urine (about 7−10 days) because starting it too early could cause very unpleasant "instant/acute withdrawal" symptoms, which no one wants or needs to happen to them. However, it can be started (safely administered) to patients either still consuming or actively withdrawing from alcohol. The author usually gives a test dose of 25 mg the first 1−3 days to see if the medication is well tolerated. If no serious side effects occur, the author then increases the dose to 50 mg each day thereafter. (In clinical trials, doses to 150 mg/day or higher have been used.) This medication has also been found to last for 2−3 days if two to three, 50 mg tabs are taken at one time,

especially on weekends. Nevertheless, in the author's experience, however, oral naltrexone therapy has been somewhat disappointing in that it is prone to discontinuation during the first 6 months of treatment in addition to the fact that patients taking more than one pill at a time sometimes forget when they last took them—which again places them at increased risk for relapse.

The author personally does not use the alternative, injectable form of extended-release naltrexone (Vivitrol) in his treatment facility despite evidence that it may be superior to oral naltrexone. The reasons are its high cost, the fact that not all insurers will totally pay for it, and most of the patients are young adults and very active physically. Thus, although this injectable medication has recently been shown, in a small study, to be very helpful in increasing the rate of patient treatment retention, it cannot be quickly removed from the body. Because this drug blocks opiate receptors and if one has an accident or breaks a bone, it may be much more difficult to expeditiously stop any accompanying pain. The pill variety will, on the other hand, only produce clinical effects in the body for about 24 h.

Vivitrol (extended-release naltrexone) is usually given IM in a 380 mg/month dose. All forms of naltrexone are nonaddicting and can be used lifelong. It has already been FDA approved for treatment of alcohol (both decreased risk of dependence behaviors and binge drinking) or opiate addiction or dependence. It should not be used in pregnancy or in nursing mothers. It can affect liver function and should not be used by those with serious liver problems (acute hepatitis, hepatic failure), so liver chemistries should be watched. The common side effects that the author has seen are temporary insomnia, headache, dizziness, nausea, and abdominal pain/diarrhea.

Medication cost without insurance:
ReVia pills—50 mg, 30 tablets $120.25
Vivitrol injection, $1630.00

ACAMPROSATE (CAMPRAL)

This medication, a GABA receptor agonist and synthetic amino acid, which is also nonaddicting, is approved as a first-line medication by the American Psychiatric Association and FDA for alcohol use disorder for extended and/or long-term use. It is most often used at this time for decreasing alcohol dependence, alleviating cravings, or maintaining abstinence. It is thought to stabilize the chemical balance in the brain (GABA vs. glutamate), which can be disrupted by alcohol (or other chemicals/substances), causing brain toxicity. It is given as a pill (666 mg) three times per day. It should be started as soon as 5 days after completion of alcohol

withdrawal as it does not appear to work if it is first taken when a patient is still drinking. The author generally uses 333 mg three times per day for 3—4 days and then increase the dose to the FDA-approved 666 mg TID. A lower dosage is sometimes effective. It has, in some clinical trials, been shown to effectively prevent alcohol use relapse, but in others, it has not been shown to be superior to either baclofen or Topamax. The dose may also need to be adjusted in patients with liver disease and *not* given to patients with severe kidney disorders (renal impairment, <30 mL/min) as it can affect renal function. Thus, a creatinine level should be obtained and reviewed before starting this medication. This medication can also cause irregular heartbeat or blood pressure changes. The somewhat common side effect that the author usually sees is diarrhea, but headaches, insomnia, or sexual side effects have also been noted. It can be used with naltrexone or cautiously in patients with liver disease.

Medication cost without insurance:
Pills (333 mg), 30 tablets $85.00

Disulfiram (Antabuse)

Disulfiram is an older medication, discovered in the 1920s and approved at the end of the 1940s, which is the original therapeutic agent used to treat chronic alcoholism by preventing the accumulation of a toxic component of alcohol. It does not reduce or stop cravings. The medication breaks down alcohol metabolites and should only be used to promote complete abstinence, which must be understood and agreed to by the patient. It appears to work best when used in a supervised treatment mode where the goal of the patient is to remain abstinent. It can begin to work within 10—30 min and produce a feeling of acute illness, withdrawal/hangover/unpleasant, and adverse side effects when alcohol is ingested within 12 h after using this medication. It is contraindicated with severe myocardial disease, coronary occlusion, or severe hepatic impairment. Monitor liver enzymes at baseline, 2 weeks later, monthly for the first 6 months, and every 3 months thereafter. While on this prescription drug and using alcohol during this time, other very unpleasant reactions can occur including increased heart rate, vomiting, nausea, headache, and confusion. Unfortunately, these very unpleasant reactions can continue for many hours or even days thereafter. Longer-term hepatic and other effects are also described in the medical literature.

Antabuse has also been used for counteracting cocaine dependence.

The author's usual dose, although rarely used, because in his experience most patients stop using it after their first bout of unpleasant side effects due to fear of a second severe reaction, is up to 500 mg each day for the first 2 weeks and then 250 mg twice per day.

Medication cost without insurance:
Pills: 250 mg, 30 tablets $199.46

NON—FDA—APPROVED LONG-TERM ANTICRAVING MEDICATIONS

Baclofen (Lioresal)

Originally designed as a muscle relaxant or central nervous system depressant to reduce spasticity from neurologic disorders, this GABA-B receptor agonist medication (it inhibits dopaminergic neurons) has already proven useful as an anticraving supplement for alcohol (especially for withdrawal in patients with advanced liver disease or heavy drinkers, but not binge drinkers) or cocaine. In fact, patients who have used this medication report becoming disinterested in the substance and thus lose their desire to use it any more. The author uses it in 20 mg doses three times per day and increases based on the patient's clinical response up to 275 mg. It appears safe for patients with liver disease. However, because of its potential central nervous system side effects (most commonly drowsiness, dizziness, decrease in mental alertness, and headache, in the author's experience), the author uses only 10 mg three times per day for 4 or so days to give the body time to adjust to or recover from these usually short-lasting issues. This medication should not be used in pregnant or breastfeeding women. It can be used for long periods of time, but it must be tapered slowly when being stopped as it can produce withdrawal symptoms. The author often uses it in combination with naltrexone. It is excreted through the kidney, so be careful in patients with renal impairment.

Medication cost without insurance:
Pills (20 mg), 30 tablets $84.20

Topiramate (Topamax)

This drug was originally designed as a medication for anticonvulsant, bipolar disorder, migraine control, and now in combination with Phentermine for weight reduction. However, it has also been found useful, off- label, to curb cravings and risk of relapse from alcohol, cocaine, and methamphetamines. It is said to reduce the number of heavy-drinking days in alcoholics at high doses (250—300 mg/day). The author usually starts at 25 mg twice per day of the immediate-release formulation for the first week and then increases to 25 mg three times per day if well tolerated, and this can be increased to 300 mg/day in 25—50 mg/week increases in two divided doses if tolerated. The extended-release formulation is contraindicated for use in alcohol consumption. It is nonaddicting but should not be used in pregnancy or in breastfeeding women. In addition, patients with a creatinine clearance <70, use no more than 50% of the usual dose. Topiramate carries a small risk of possible suicidal behavior or thoughts, confusion, memory problems, sleepiness, paresthesia, or ability to concentrate. The side effects that the author has most commonly seen include sleepiness, dizziness, nausea, cold-like symptoms, and diarrhea. Blurred vision or eye pain should cause a patient to see an eye doctor. It can be started after alcohol withdrawal, but the author only begins using it 7—10 days after stopping opiates or uppers (cocaine or methamphetamines), as many people often become temporarily very tired due to short-term brain chemical alterations when use of any substances is discontinued. It should not be stopped suddenly but tapered slowly.

Medication cost without insurance:
Pills: 25 mg, 30 tablets $599.84

Gabapentin (Neurontin)

An NIH-funded study has noted promising results from the use of gabapentin for alcohol dependence treatment after naltrexone and acamprosate failure. The most positive results were obtained with an 1800 mg dose given as 600 mg TID. However, it needs to be titrated slowly starting at 300 mg and increased in 300 mg/day increments. These patients proved to be twice as likely to refrain from heavy drinking (cravings) and four times as likely to stop drinking altogether. It was also found to improve sleep and mood stabilization in this group of patients. The medication was found to be well tolerated with few side effects. Common side effects include dizziness, fatigue, visual disturbances, and uncommon psychotic-like behavior. Please remember that gabapentin is a potentially harmful and misused drug as it is often consumed for recreational purposes and self-medication. It is said to also potentiate the effects of other substances when used in combination with them. Be very careful in elderly patients.

Medication cost without insurance:
Pills: 300 mg, 30 pills, $15.00

Ondansetron (Zofran)

Originally developed as an antiemetic agent, because it reduces serotonin-mediated dopaminergic effects, it also demonstrated to be effective in alcohol-induced gratification, total days of abstinence and consumption. It is interesting that studies using this medication were most effective in patients who started drinking after age 25. Clinical benefits from this drug usually occur at a dose between 0.001 and 0.016 mg/kg BID, but the medication has been successful to 2 mg BID. (Because the medication only comes in 4 and 8 mg tabs, one must use 2 mg BID.) Common side effects include fatigue, headache, anxiety, and serotonin syndrome (if used with other serotonin-producing agents). Monitor patients with an electrolyte imbalance using an ECG.

Medication cost without insurance:
4 mg, 30 tablets—$60.00

OTHER MEDICATIONS
Varenicline (Chantix)
This medication as previously noted is an effective smoking cessation drug because of its effect on the nicotine receptor and appears to possibly be a mediator of craving control for other abused substances. Recent investigation has now shown that this medication decreases heavy-drinking days, especially in men. Thus, as the relationship between smoking and alcohol consumption continues to grow, this medication should be considered more often.

Medication cost without insurance: $503.00

Pregabalin (Lyrica)
This medication has recently been reported to help with alcohol addiction due to its positive effects on the GABA neurotransmitter pathway. However, it is a controlled medication as it is said to have an addiction potential and is very expensive at this time because it is nongeneric. The author has not tried it on any of his patients.

Medication cost without insurance is about $4: 50—4:75 per pill.

Nalmefene (Selincro)
For completeness, this medication is used in Europe for alcohol and gambling disorders but is not approved in the United States at this time for substance abuse disorders (although originally approved in the United States for opioid overdose but was then taken off the market due to poor sales). It is similar in structure to naltrexone and has a half-life somewhere between naloxone and naltrexone.

Common Substance Abuse—Associated Sexually Transmitted Diseases

INTRODUCTION

The incidence of certain microbial diseases (bacterial, viral, parasite) is markedly increased in the substance abuse population. Many causes have been recognized including increased high-risk sexual behaviors, poor hygiene, and sharing contaminated household products, substances, and needles. Finally, impaired immune defenses by various mechanisms also appear to play a role.

In addition to the diseases discussed in this chapter, other microbial infections of concern in drug users include injection-related skin infections, aspiration pneumonia secondary to alterations in consciousness from the substances used, endocarditis (heart infection), septic emboli, and bone and joint infections due to hematogenous (blood) pathogen dissemination.

All of the disorders discussed below appear to have a latent/subclinical or asymptomatic period of varying lengths during which transmission from infected to unknowing, noninfected individuals often occurs. Patients may also be infected by more than one STD-causing organism at any one time. Treatment and partner notification, often through intervention by the local or state health departments, are also an integral part of this process to prevent potential reinfection and/or suspension of further transmission.

This section briefly discusses some of the common sexually transmitted diseases (STDs) and tuberculosis. Also included are helpful risk factor screening, testing, appropriate counseling, health department consulting, updated information for teaching the substance abuse population, and initial clinical management information for health professionals who deal with this population. Finally, it is important that all healthcare professionals know, in the author's opinion, this current and correct information, due to the large number of misconceptions often expressed by substance abuse patients during his discussions with them (and other members of the treatment team).

The American Public Health Association has published the following general guidelines to reduce STD transmission:

a. Use condom unless you are recently tested clear and/or monogamous
b. Get tested if an STD is suspected
c. Get treated if you have an STD
d. Initiate expedited partner therapy (EPD)

This involves immediately telling your partner about your STD before intimacy to prevent possible "surprise" transmission and enable them to be promptly evaluated and/or treated if necessary. In addition, the use/notification of the local health department is especially important to help with treatment, follow-up, and possible treatment of sexual contacts.

It is important to note that treatment for these diseases will not be emphasized in this chapter because recommendations from the Centers for Disease Control continually change over time. For a more complete discussion on each individual disease and its treatment, see https://www.cdc.gov/nchhstp/atlas/.

Human Immunodeficiency Virus

The human immunodeficiency virus (HIV) affects (attacks) the immune system, and immunodeficiency is the cornerstone of all the manifestations of this disease.

HIV infection was initially considered a fatal disease as we had no way to stop its progression to AIDS in the United States, but now, with the advent of new treatment medications (e.g., retroviral therapy) capable of markedly reducing the viral load, it is now generally characterized as a chronic illness because most who are currently affected usually enjoy a normal life span.

Modes of transmission are similar to hepatitis B with respect to certain sexual practices with infected partners. This includes oral sex, male to male anal sex, multiple sex partners, blood to blood transmission, needle sticks with an infected needle, unsafe sexual behaviors (sex with HIV-infected person), shared needles, or heterosexual

Addiction Medicine for Health Care Professionals. https://doi.org/10.1016/B978-0-323-68017-2.00006-5

vaginal sex. Male circumcision has been found to be helpful in prevention of this disease.

The African-American population has been disproportionately hard hit by this disease. In addition, people with HIV can remain asymptomatic for years (sometimes as much as 10) before clinical manifestations occur.

HIV screening should be routinely conducted on all substance abusers unless legal restraints interfere. However, screening is not always useful early in the disease process as the incubation period can be up to 6 months before it becomes positive. In addition, despite significant advances in HIV detection, the CDC has reported that in 2015, approximately 15% of HIV cases are still unreported with the delay between infection and diagnosis of 2 years for women who injected drugs and 4.9 years for heterosexual men, 2.2 years among whites, and 4.2 years among Asians.

HIV often begins with nonspecific symptoms such as weight loss, infection, and fever. It can affect every organ and cause cancers. Pregnant women with HIV should deliver by C-section and not breastfeed.

Currently no vaccine exists to prevent HIV. Thus, prevention of HIV depends on HIV screening, testing, counseling, prudent sexual practices, and cessation of injectable drug use. Thus, **safe sex and safe and sterile needle use to prevent exchange of body fluids are especially important for the substance abuse population**.

If exposed during the occurrence of a sexual assault, incest, inadvertent sex with an infected partner, or a pregnancy in an HIV-affected individual, the use of antiretroviral therapy may be helpful in preventing this disease in the affected person, sexual partner, or the developing fetus.

Written consent for testing may be required in some states.

Those who test positive, as is the case with all STDs, should be referred to a physician specializing in this area of medicine or a local or state health department to be connected to ongoing medical care, including obtaining a viral load evaluation and partner notification services.

Treatment is directed at decreasing the amount of virus in the blood (viral load) to zero (or as close as possible).

Newer medications or medication combinations are currently being developed and incorporated into treatment regimens.

Hepatitis

Hepatitis can be caused by five, so far identified, viruses, in addition to many drugs and toxic agents. In this brief discussion, we will only concentrate on this disorder caused by the viruses hepatitis A, B, and C. It should also be noted that the liver chemistry test alanine aminotransferase (ALT) is usually the first to rise (4—12 weeks) when liver injury occurs. In addition, without getting too technical, an elevated immunoglobulin IgM level indicates a positive diagnosis, and an elevated IgG level is associated with immunity to the virus. Vaccination may be helpful as a prophylaxis measure in preventing postexposure hepatitis A and/or B.

Hepatitis A

Often called infectious hepatitis, it is most often spread by the fecal-oral route from someone coming into contact with fecal material from an individual with this disease.

It is also prone to dissemination (possibly rapid) in areas of the world characterized by crowded conditions where there is also poor sanitation and direct contact with infected persons. It can additionally occur from contaminated water or food, especially inadequately cooked shellfish and from adopted children arriving from other countries. Furthermore, it has been reported in people who inject contaminated drugs, men who have sex with men, people with chronic liver disease, and those with blood clotting disorders.

Hepatitis A virus (HAV) has an incubation period of approximately 30 days, and it is can be found in feces for up to 2 weeks before people start to show symptoms. There is often accompanying nausea, vomiting, weakness, decreased appetite, and an aversion to smoking. Affected individuals characteristically have a swollen, tender liver and/or jaundice (yellowing of the skin and eyes), and elevated liver chemistries.

It is usually more severe in adults than children, in whom it usually occurs without symptoms.

The illness usually subsides within 2—3 weeks but can reoccur. Recovery is usually complete within 3 months.

Prevention is best accomplished by handwashing after bowel movement.

There is now a vaccine to prevent this virus that can be given to both children and adults. In fact, children under 1 year of age are now given this vaccine as an infant and a second dose within the next 6—12 months, plus those who are at increased risk for the infection or for complications from HAV.

Hepatitis B

This virus is usually transmitted through infected blood, sharing needles by drug users, incarcerated individuals, and hepatitis B virus (HBV)-infected contacts but can also be transmitted by sex as the virus is present in saliva, semen, and vaginal secretions. Untreated HVB patients have a 15%–40% chance of developing cirrhosis, which may then lead to liver failure and liver cancer.

The incubation period for this virus is 6 weeks to 6 months.

In this country, all children are (or should be) immunized against hepatitis B starting at birth.

HBV infection usually starts in a manner similar to that of hepatitis A. In those not immunized (usually this is performed as an infant), it can lead to severe/chronic liver disease, liver transplantation and/or possibly liver cancer, and death (hepatitis B is responsible for up to 80% of hepatocellular carcinoma). Hepatitis B surface antigen (HBsAg) is usually the first test to become abnormal with active Hep-B and usually appears before clinical symptoms appear. Elevated levels of this antigen continue to appear in the carrier state or with chronic active hepatitis. Hepatitis B surface antibody (HBsAb) generally appears about 1 month after the disappearance of the surface antigen and indicates that the acute infection phase has passed and notes immunity to further Hep-B infection. This antibody also becomes positive after Hep-B vaccine immunization. Hepatitis B core antibody (HBcAb) starts to appear after 1 month of Hep-B infection and may be present for years. It is usually considered as a marker of recent hepatitis infection. Other B hepatitis markers may be present but are beyond the scope of this book.

The FDA has recently warned of the risk of HBV reactivation in patients coinfected with hepatitis C virus (HCV)—both before and after HCV treatment. The reason for this warning is because HCV infection is thought to suppress HBV replication. Once HCV has been eradicated, however, HBV viral replication may then reactivate. This warning includes the following:

1. All patients with evidence of current or prior HBV infection should be tested for evidence of rapid HBV DNA replication in addition to their HCV viral load/HCV RNA infestation blood test. Reactivation has been found by measuring HBsAg, indicating that they are currently HBV positive, and even patients who have a positive hepatitis core antibody (anti-HBc), which usually indicates a resolved HBV infection, are actually now positive again due to the reappearance of the HBsAg. This testing must be performed before initiating treatment with HCV direct-acting antiviral agents (DDAs).
2. Patients with serologic evidence of HBV infection should be monitored for clinical or laboratory signs of a hepatitis B flare-up (increased or increasing liver chemistries, jaundice) or HBV reactivation during HCV treatment and also during posttreatment follow-up.
3. Appropriate patient management for HBV should be initiated when clinically indicated by physicians skilled in hepatitis management.
4. A recent scientific article indicates that consumption of at least three cups of coffee daily was tied to a reduction in all-cause mortality among patients with HBV/HCV and HCV/HIV coinfections.
5. All patients with chronic HBV infections should be monitored for hepatocellular carcinoma. HBV is said to have a low cure rate with appropriate medication, but progression of the disease can be prevented indefinitely by long-term treatment using these same medications.

Hepatitis C

Unfortunately, only 25% of those affected with HCV have been diagnosed to date, and only 9% have been treated. HCV is more common in males and non-Hispanic black population.

In 2007, HCV patients died at a mean age of 57 years. This is 20 years shorter than the average US life span. In that year, HCV mortality rate surpassed the HIV mortality rate. Almost 20,000 people died in the United States in 2014 due to chronic HCV infection.

Over 50% of cases are found in people who share needles (not those who use needles but do not share them with others). Reinfection can also occur.

Other common causes are sharing body fluids, often by the use of unclean instruments when tattooing, body piercing or concurrent HIV infection, high-risk sexual behaviors, incarceration, product sharing such as a tooth brush, intranasal illicit drug use, hemodialysis, blood transfusion before 1992, and being born to an HCV-positive mother.

Lastly, HCV infection is considered to be at heightened risk/prevalence in people born between 1945 and 1965, regardless of risk factors as it is thought that 75% of chronic HCV infections can be found in this group of people.

It is less commonly transmitted by sexual contact than hepatitis B except in those with multiple partners (both heterosexual and same sex relationships) and who engage in unprotected sex.

Acute HCV infection is generally asymptomatic. The incubation period of this disease is about 6–7 weeks, and some of those infected (about 30%) are able to destroy this virus with their own body immunity. Thus, those found to have a positive hepatitis C antibody test need to have a viral load for HCV-RNA viral count obtained to determine if the virus has or has not been destroyed by their own body immunity. HCV genotyping may also be ordered (70% of those with hepatitis C have type 1 genotype, and 20% have type 2 genotype), in addition to a CBC, kidney and liver function testing. In these patients who spontaneously clear the virus, no additional testing is necessary unless they were recently reexposed, as it can recur, when repeat HCV testing can be considered again in 6 months.

Patients with chronic HCV infections should also be tested for HAV, HIV, and HBV infection and offered pneumococcal vaccinations.

It is important to note that those who are able to spontaneously destroy the HCV will still remain positive for the HCV antibody for the rest of their life (but have no positive viral load).

Chronic hepatitis C progresses slowly (with often a decade or two of no clinical activity) but will usually occur in about 75%–85% of those who had acute hepatitis C. Chronic HCV infection can lead to liver failure, liver cancer, and death. Twenty percent will develop cirrhosis within 20 years of diagnosis. In fact hepatitis C is the leading cause of liver transplantation and liver cancer although nonalcoholic steatohepatitis/nonalcoholic fatty liver disease is rapidly increasing as a cause of liver cancer.

Until recently, the treatment/control of hepatitis C was only fair at best. However, today it is almost 100% curable with the medications now available.

The current drugs work quickly and are well tolerated with only few side effects (nausea, headache, fatigue, itching insomnia, and weakness were most commonly reported).

All those with a positive hepatitis C antibody test and who still have the presence of the virus in their blood, regardless of clinical symptoms, should be referred to a hepatitis specialist (usually an infectious disease physician or gastroenterologist) who can follow them long term and recommend further treatment at the appropriate time.

Human Papillomavirus

Human papillomavirus (HPV) is the most common sexually transmitted infection in the United States. It is a well-described virus, with well over 100 types, capable of causing multiple cancers, including the cervix, anus, vocal chords, nose, and most commonly seen venereal (genital) warts, which is considered a non–cancer-forming STD. Most cases of HPV are spread by mouth, skin, and genital contact but are most often cleared by the body's immune system or most strains are not potentially cancer producing.

Concerning its cancer-forming ability, 70% of cervical cancer is caused by types 16 and 18. Ninety percent of genital warts are caused by types 6 and 11. The National Center for Health Statistics (NCHS) has recently reported that more than 40% of adults in the United States have been exposed to HPV.

Genital warts have a long incubation period which averages 2–18 months. Sometimes they are cured spontaneously but can also recur. Multiple treatments are available to temporarily "cure" these warts but are often painful. They can usually be diagnosed by your physician on inspection and, as noted above, usually are not associated with cancer.

A vaccine now exists to prevent certain types of these warts or cancers. The vaccine incorporates/targets nine HPV types 6, 11, 16, 18, 31, 33, 45, 52, and 58. This vaccine thus acts to prevent infection with the most common viral strains causing these warts and 90% of the cancers including cervical, anal, oropharyngeal, vaginal, and vulvar. Cervical cancer, according to the CDC, is the fourth leading cause of cancer worldwide in women, and oral cancer has become more common than nicotine-induced cancer in males.

The vaccine is FDA approved for use in children before they become sexually active or can become infected but is also effective in adults (ages 9–45 for males and females) but can be considered at any time during one's life to protect them from the strains, which they have not already acquired (have not already become infected with). In fact, a new study indicates that a nonavalent HPV vaccination by age 9 may reduce cervical cancer by 76%. As recommended by the Advisory Committee on Immunization Practices, as noted in the reference section for STDs, it is usually given in a two- to three-dose schedule.

Circumcision is also an HPV deterrent.

The vaccine is moderately expensive and thus underused (at this time, only 40% of teenage girls and 25% of teenage boys have been immunized). In the past, three immunizations were recommended, but only two doses are now found to be effective in teenagers. In women, cotesting for cervical HPV infection is sometimes recommended with routine pap smears.

Herpes Viral Infections

Two strains of herpes viral infections are considered to be part of the STD infection group. These include herpes simplex (herpes 1) or cold, canker, or fever sores of the lips and mouth area and herpes genitalis (herpes 2), or genital/sexual herpes.

a. Herpes 1 infection

It usually causes painful blisters on the lips or in the mouth area.

It can occur from virus shed from infected but either symptomatic or asymptomatic individual by kissing or other forms of contact and can recur.

The initial infection is usually more painful than recurrences.

Recurrent infection generally heals faster than the primary one.

It generally forms an ulcer if not treated within 1–2 weeks.

Herpes 1 infection can also cause blisters in the genital region.

Multiple antiviral medications are now available to treat, but not cure this infection.

b. Herpes 2 infection

Usually causes painful blisters and later ulcers in the genital area, anal area, buttocks, or upper thighs.

In women, cervical pain, urination difficulty, or urine retention often occurs.

Recurrence is common.

Most people are unaware that they are affected despite the painful blisters.

Besides antiviral medications, circumcision and condom barrier protection are extremely important in preventing disease spread.

Disclosure to sexual partners is associated with a 50% reduction in herpes 2 acquisition.

Diagnostic blood testing is not advised. In addition, results of a reported positive herpes 2 infection should not be interpreted in asymptomatic individuals, as recently published by the CDC.

Gonorrhea—A Sexually Transmitted Disease Caused by a Bacterium

Gonorrhea, colloquially known as the clap is usually transmitted by sexual activity. It has an incubation period of 2–8 days.

It appears to be most common in the 15- to 29-year-old group.

In men it usually causes an infected, large yellowish/creamy-looking penile discharge with burning on urination.

This disease often involves the prostate and other internal male glands.

In women, symptoms are usually worse during menses with urinary problems and a discharge from the urinary tract and vagina.

Anal involvement can occur.

Urinary culture or urinary DNA testing is recommended for identification.

Antibiotic treatment is the usual method of therapy. Please refer to the newest FDA/CDC recommendations.

It should be noted, however, that gonorrhea is now becoming more antibiotic resistant.

It is recommended that both the infected patient and sexual partners also be tested for syphilis and HIV.

Chlamydia

This disease is caused by a parasite similar to a bacterium called *Chlamydia trachomatis*. It is also called lymphogranuloma venereum.

The strains of this parasite which can cause the sexually transmitted form of this infection, are usually spread through direct contact with the infected/active genital sore.

The incubation period is 5–21 days and often goes unnoticed.

The disease is capable of spreading to the lymph glands, which become enlarged, soft, and start to drain in the groin and rectal areas.

In men, if the original blister or ulcer is not noticed, it will cause swollen lymph glands in the groin, which then often open and start to drain (buboes).

In women, if the discharge is initially unnoticed in the urethra or cervix, it then drains via the lymph to the anal region and anal glands where an infected discharge occurs.

Late manifestations include proctitis and rectal stricture.

Urine DNA testing is used to detect this parasite.

Treatment is by antibiotics as recommended by the CDC.

Trichomoniasis

Trichomoniasis (Trich) is one of the most common STDs. In the United States, in 2015, 122 million cases were diagnosed. It is caused by a single-cell parasite and transmitted through sex or touching (vaginal, oral, or anal). It is interesting that many of those infected, especially men, do not have symptoms of this infection. Condom use is very helpful for prevention.

If symptoms appear, they often start 5–28 days after exposure. Most often, there is itching or pain in the genital area, vaginal discharge, burning on urination, and pain with sex. Screening for trichomoniasis is recommended for women with HIV, as this disease increases the risk of transmitting HIV to the fetus.

Diagnosis is best using urine nucleic amplification testing, and this disease is treated with antibiotic therapy.

Syphilis

Syphilis is caused by a parasite called spirochete.

Most commonly it is transmitted by unprotected sex (including oral sex). Reexposure after successful treatment can also occur.

It is capable of affecting any organ of the body.

It generally occurs in two stages. The first stage is typically characterized by a painless ulcer about 3–4 weeks after infection on the penis and genital area in men, or vagina and genital area in women. The ulcers can also occur in the rectum, throat, tongue, lip, or wherever contact was made.

The disease then goes into a dormant period until, in the second phase, it spreads throughout the body. It can eventually cause serious disability or death, especially if it attacks the brain (neurosyphilis).

Syphilis is common among HIV-affected patients, and HIV testing is appropriate/prudent for all patients infected with syphilis.

Diagnosis (both screening and definitive testing) is best performed by serologic testing. Thus, it is often a two-test process as positive screening tests must be confirmed by definitive testing before treatment should be recommended. Follow-up testing is also important (at 6 and 12 months after treatment). Positive testing should include contact with local or state health departments to aid in treatment and follow-up help in detection of other possible concurrent STD infections, and identification, evaluation, and possibly treatment of infected sexual partners.

It is treated with antibiotics, especially long-acting penicillin, which kills all the infecting parasites and stops the disease from inflicting further body damage. Differing amounts of antibiotics may be needed when the length of the latent period is unknown.

A discussion of tertiary syphilis is beyond the scope of this book.

Tuberculosis

This disease is the leading cause of worldwide infectious disease mortality (approximately 5000 people per day), and thus it is considered a very severe public health crisis.

It is caused by a bacterium (*Mycobacterium tuberculosis*). It is said to infect about one-third of the world's population, including an estimated 11 million people in the United States. Only about 5%–10% of those infected develop active tuberculosis (TB) during their lifetime.

It most commonly occurs in areas where disadvantaged populations live. These areas are characterized by those who are malnourished and homeless, who must live in overcrowded and often substandard housing or on the street. It also occurs disproportionately in the HIV-infected population and substance abuse population and should be suspected in people who have lived or recently traveled to countries where TB infection is common, may have had or been treated for TB in the past, recently spent time or had close contact with a person who had past active disease, or ever had a positive TB skin test or worked in a laboratory-handling TB bacteria.

Tuberculosis is spread by inhalation of a droplet of sputum into a susceptible individual from an infected person. The disease will occur if the normal body immunity is unable to contain and destroy the organisms inhaled.

Once established in the body, it begins to spread. This is called the primary infection or latent tuberculosis infection, as the body is now only able to contain, but not destroy the organisms. The disease can later be reactivated at any time if the body's immune defenses become impaired in any way. The primary infection has no clinical or radiologic manifestations.

During the latent period of the primary infection, this disease is not active and cannot be transmitted to others unless there is an immune system problem where reactivation can recur. During this period, the disease can be properly treated with preventive antibiotic therapy medications/drugs. Latent TB can become active without appropriate treatment.

TB treatment usually takes at least 6 months, which often promotes noncompliance. Recent scientific studies have indicated that one possible reason for the difficulty in quickly being able to eradicate TB infection may be due to the organism's ability to shift its metabolism to another metabolic pathway, which allows it to continue living, but one in which the antibiotics used will not work successfully.

If not properly or fully treated, or due to an inadequate immune response, progressive primary tuberculosis will develop. Development of this stage will now affect the lungs and other body organs in a clinically recognizable manner.

An infected person will usually show symptoms of chronic illness including malaise, weight loss, anorexia, night sweats, and fever. However, the most common manifestation of TB during the primary period is a chronic cough, often dry at first but slowly becoming more purulent and blood streaked.

Multiple proven laboratory or skin tests are available to diagnose this condition.

Certain criteria may be helpful in assessing whether a person should have a skin test. These include chronic cough (more than 2 weeks); coughing up blood; recent contact with a person infected with TB; immigration from a country with a high rate of TB in last 5 years; previous organ transplant; previous time in jail, nursing home, or prison; previous or present drug injection; worked in a lab that processed TB specimens; and a history of an abnormal chest X-ray.

Usually, patients with one or more of the above noted risk factors should receive a tuberculin skin test, with the Mantoux method being the most commonly used. This test uses 0.1 mL of purified protein derivative in a tuberculin syringe with a very thin needle. This test contains 5 tuberculin units which are injected under the skin on the volar/inside surface of the forearm.

The size of the red, skin induration/hardening is examined at 48–72 h, using a millimeter ruler. A positive skin test is a transverse diameter of 5 mm or more. If positive, a chest X-ray is indicated with prompt follow-up treatment by a TB specialist and/or the local or state health departments who are primarily responsible for finding, testing, and treating contacts.

Finally, for those who have no definite risks for TB testing but a physical exam possibly notes otherwise, the interferon-gamma release assay (IGRA) is recommended, with follow-up testing if positive.

References

GENERAL REFERENCES

American Pharmacists Association, 2016. Drug Information Handbook. Lexicomp, Wolters/Kluwer.

Brunton, L. (Ed.), 2016. Goodman and Gillman's the Pharmacological Basis of Therapeutics. McGraw-Hill.

Calacuiti, C.A. (Ed.), 2011. Principles of Addiction Medicine-the Essentials. Lippincott Williams and Wilkins, Wolters/Kluwer.

Inaba, D.S., Cohen, W.E., 2014. Uppers, Downers, All Arounders. CNS Productions Inc.

Papadakis, M.A. (Ed.), 2018. Current Medical Diagnosis and Treatments. McGraw-Hill.

Ries, R.K. (Ed.), 2014. The ASAM Principles of Addiction Medicine. Wolters/Kluwer.

Sydor, A., 2009. Molecular Neuropharmacology: A Foundation for Clinical Neuroscience. McGraw-Hill.

SELECTED REFERENCES

Section 1: Introduction

Ajmera, V., et al., 2018. Even modest alcohol use may worsen NAFLD. Clin. Gastroenterol. Hepatol. https://doi.org/10.1016/j.cgh.2018.01.026.

Alderks, C.E., 2017. Trends in the use of methadone, buprinorphine, and extended release naltrexone at substance abuse facilities: 2003−2015 (update). In: The CBHSQ Report Center for Behavioral Health Statistics and Quality, Substance Abuse and Mental Health Services Administration, Rockville, MD.

American Society of Addiction Medicine. Public Policy Statement: Definition of Addiction 4/12/2011.

Argoff, C.E., et al., 2018. Rational urine drug monitoring in patients receiving opioids for chronic pain: consensus recommendations. Pain Med. 19, 97.

Astarita, G., Avanesian, A., et al., 2015. Methamphetamine accelerates cellular senescence through stimulation of de novo ceramide biosynthesis. PLoS One 10 (2), e0116961. https://doi.org/10.1371/journal.pone.0116961.

Baeulieu, J.M., Gainetdinov, R.R., 2011. The physiology, signaling, and pharmacology of dopamine receptors. Pharmacol. Rev. 63, 182.

Bilinski, P., et al., 2012. Epigenetic regulation in drug addiction. Ann. Agric. Environ. Med. 19, 491.

Blevins, E.C., et al., 2018. Gaps in the substance use disorder treatment referral process: provider perceptions. J. Addict. Med. 12, 273.

Blum, K., et al., 2012. Sex, drugs, and rock and roll: hypothesizing common mesolimbic activation as a function of reward gene polymorphisms. J. Psychoactive Drugs 44, 38.

Bonnie, R.J., et al., 2017. Both urgency and balance needed in addressing opioid epidemic: a report from the National Academies of Sciences, Engineering, and Medicine. JAMA 318, 423.

Broussard, J.I., 2012. Co-transmission of dopamine and glutamate. J. Gen. Physiol. 139, 93.

Bunken, R., et al., 2017. Abuse-deterrent Formulations of Opioids: Effectiveness and Value. Institute for Clinical and Economic Review. https//icer-review.org/wp-content/uploads/2016/08/NECEPAC_Final_Report_08_08_17.pdf.

CDC, 2017. Characteristics of initial prescription episodes and likelihood of long-term opioid use-United States, 2006−2015. Weekly 66 (10), 265.

Dunne, E.M., et al., 2015. Increased risk for substance abuse and health related problems among homeless veterans. Am. J. Addict. 24, 676.

Dwyer-Lundgren, l, et al., 2018. Trends and patterns of geographic variation in mortality from substance use disorders and intentional injuries among US counties. JAMA 319, 1013.

Ersche, K.D., et al., 2017. Disrupted iron regulation in the brain and periphery in cocaine addiction. Transl. Psychiatry 7, e1040. https://doi.org/10.10-38/tp.2016.271.

Frank, J.W., et al., 2017. Patient outcomes in dose reduction or discontinuation of long-term opioid therapy: a systematic review. Ann. Intern. Med. 167, 181.

Fratta, W., Fattore, L., 2013. Molecular mechanisms of cannabinoid addiction. Curr. Opin. Neurobiol. 23, 487.

Friemel, C.M., Zimmer, A., Schneider, M., 2014. The CB1 receptor as an important mediator of hedonic reward processing. Neuropsychopharmacology 39, 2387.

Giardino, W.J., et al., 2018. Parallel circuits from the bed nuclei of stria terminalis to the lateral hypothalamus drive opposing emotional states. Nat. Neurosci. 21, 1084.

Gottlieb, S., 2017. Support for treating opioid addiction with medication. JAMA 318, 2071.

Grant, B.F., et al., 2017. Prevalence of 12 month alcohol use, high−risk drinking, and DSM-1V alcohol use disorder in the United States, 2001−2002 to 2012−2013. Results from the national epidemiologic survey on alcohol and related conditions. JAMA Psychiatry. https://doi.org/10.1001/jamapsychiatry.2017.2161.

Hampton, T., et al., 2018. Scientists separate opioid's analgesic effects from their dangerous respiratory effects. JAMA 319, 855.

Hampton, T., 2018. Research reveals mechanism that may drive alcohol use disorder. JAMA 320, 862.

Hawker, G.A., et al., 2011. Measures of adult pain. Arthritis Care Res. (Hoboken) 211 (63), S240.

Henry, S.G., et al., 2015. Dose escalation during the first year of long term opioid therapy for chronic pain. Pain Med. 16, 733.

Hoggatt, K.J., et al., 2017. Prevalence of substance misuse among US veterans in the general population. J. Addict. Med. https://doi.org/10.1111/ajad.12534. PMID: 28370701.

Jardine, W.P., Hassan, Y.A.A., 2014. Multiple and substitute addictions involving prescription drugs misuse among 12th graders: gateway theory revisited with market basket analysis. J. Addict. Med. https://doi.org/10.1097/ADM.000 0000000000012.

Jonan, A.B., et al., 2018. Buprinorphine formulations: clinical best practice strategies recommendations for perioperative management of patients undergoing surgical or interventional pain procedures. Pain Physician 21 (1), E1–E12. PMID: 29357325.

Jones, T., et al., 2012. A comparison of various screening methods in predicting discharge from opiate treatment. Clin. J. Pain 28, 93.

Jordan, C.J., Andersen, S.L., 2016. Sensitive periods of substance abuse: early risk for transition to dependence. Dev. Cogn. Neurosci. https://doi.org/10.10101016/j.den.2016.10.004.

Koh, H.K., 2017. Community-based prevention and strategies for the opioid crisis. JAMA 318, 993.

Krebs, E.E., et al., 2018. Effect of opioid vs nonopioid medications on pain-related function in patients with chronic back pain or hip or knee osteoarthritis pain: the SPACE randomized clinical trial. JAMA 319, 872.

Kurdyak, P., Rehm, J., 2012. High toll of mental illness and addictions must be addressed. Psycho. Psych. http://medicalxpress.com/news/2-12-10-high-toll-mental-illness-addictions.html.

Lemmon, R., Hampton, A., 2018. Nonpharmacologic treatment of chronic pain: what works. J. Fam. Pract. 67, 474.

Manchikanti, L., et al., 2017. Responsible, safe and effective prescription of opioids for non-cancer pain: American Society for Interventional Pain Physicians (ASIPP) guidelines. Pain Physician 20, S3.

Marino-Lopez, L., Stamatakis, E.A., et al., 2012. Neural correlates of severity of cocaine, heroin, alcohol, MDMA, and cannabis use in polysubstance abusers: a resting-PET brain metabolism study. PLoS One 7.

Mole, B., 2017. With a 10 Day Supply of Opioids, 1 in 5 Become Long Term Users. http://arstechnica.com/science/2017/03/.

National Academy of Sciences Engineering and Medicine, 2017. The Health Effects of Cannabis and Cannabinoids: The Current State of Evidence and Recommendations for Research. The National Academies Press, Washington DC.

Nestler, E.J., 2012. Transcriptional mechanisms of drug addiction. Clin. Psychopharmacol. Neurosci. 10, 136.

Nestler, E.J., 2013. Cellular basis of memory for addiction. Dialogues. Clin. Neurosci. 15, 431.

Nestler, E.J., 2014. Epigenetic mechanisms of drug addiction. Neuropharmacology 76, 259.

NIDA Researchers Confirm Important Brain Reward Pathway, 2014. http://www.nih.gov/news/health/nov2014/nida-htm.

Nutt, D.J., et al., 2015. The dopamine theory of addiction: 40 years of highs and lows. Nat. Rev. Neurosci. 16, 305.

Okasanya, A., Li, X., 2018. Loperamide abuse and dependence; clinical features and treatment considerations. J. Addict. Med. 12, 496.

Oliveto, A., Gentry, W.B., et al., 2010. Behavioral effects of gamma-hydroxybutyrate in humans. Behav. Pharmacol. 21, 332.

Olsen, Y., Scharfstein, J.M., 2014. Confronting the stigma of opiate use disorder-and its treatment. JAMA. https://doi.org/10.100/jama.2014.2147. Published Online 2/26/14.

Olsen, C.M., 2011. Natural rewards, neuroplasticity, and non-drug addictions. Neuropharmacology 61, 1109.

Parks Thomas, C., et al., 2018. Applying American Society of Addiction Medicine Performance Measures in Commercial Health Insurance and Service Date. J. Addict. Med. 12, 287.

Peltz, G., Sudhof, T.C., 2018. The neurobiology of opioid addiction and the potential for prevention strategies. JAMA 319, 2071.

Perry, et al., 2014. Role of cues and contexts on drug seeking behavior. Brit. J. Pharmacol. 171, 4636.

Peterson, A.L., 2013. Integrating mental health and addiction services to improve clinical outcomes. Issues Mental Health Nurs. 34 (10), 752–756, e39830. https://doi.org/10.1371/journal.pone.0039830.

Pitchers, K.K., et al., 2013. Natural and drug rewards act on common neural plasticity mechanisms with delta FosB as a key mediator. J. Neurosci. 33, 3434.

Rodenberg, C., 2012. This is our society on drugs: top 5 infographics. Sci. Am. http://blogs.scientificamerican.com/white-noise/2012/04/20.

Rosenbloom, D.L., 2018. Commentary on "gaps" in the substance use disorder treatment referral process: provider perceptions. J. Addict. Med. 12, 255.

Ruffle, J.K., 2014. Molecular neurobiology of addiction: what is the deltaFosB about? Am. J. Drug Alcohol Abuse 40, 428.

Sample I Natural Painkiller Nasal Spray Could Replace Addictive Opioids, Trial Indicates, 2018. The Guardian.

Saunders, J.B., 2017. Substance use and addictive disorders in DSM-5 and ICD-10 and the draft ICD-11. Curr. Opin. Psychiatry 30, 360.

Savage, S.R., 2013. What to do when pain and addiction coexist. J. Fam. Pract. 62, S10.

Saxon, A.J., 2018. The unmet challenges of co-occurring opioid and alcohol use. Alcohol. Clin. Exp. Res. 42, 1406.

Schuchat, A., et al., 2017. New data on opioid prescribing in the United States. JAMA 318, 425.

Shah, A., et al., 2017. Characteristics of initial prescription episodes and likelihood of long term opioid use-United States, 2006–2015. MMWR Morb. Mortal. Wkly. Rep. 66, 265.

Sofuoglu, M., Rosenheck, R., 2014. Petrakis I pharmacological treatment of comorbid PTSD and substance use disorder: recent progress. Addict. Behav. 39, 428.

Stefano, G.B., et al., 2012. Endogenous morphine: up to date review. Folia Biol. (Praha) 58, 49.

Steiner, H., et al., 2013. Addiction related gene regulation: risks of exposure to cognitive enhancers vs. other psychostimulants. Prog. Neurobiol. 100, 60.

US Department of Health and Human Services Detoxification and Substance Abuse Treatment, 2006.

Vassoler, F.M., Sadri-Vakali, G., 2014. Mechanisms of transgenerational inheritance of addictive like behaviors. Neuroscience 264, 198.

Vink, J., et al., 2018. Schizophrenia and cannabis use may share common genes. Nat. Neurosci. https://doi.org/10.1038/s41593-018-0206-1.

Volkow, N.D., Koob, G.F., Mclellan, 2016. Neurobiologic advances from the brain disease model of addiction. N. Engl. J. Med 374, 363.

Walker, D.M., et al., 2015. Regulation of chromatin states bt drugs of abuse. Curr. Opin. Neurobiol. 30, 112.

Weiss, A.J., et al., Opioid Related Inpatient Stays and Emergency Department Visits by State, 2009–2014 2016 HCUP Statistical Brief #219. Agency for Healthcare Research Quality, Rockville, MD. www.hcup-us.ahrq.gov/reports/statbriefs/sb219-Opioid-Hospital-Stays-ED-Visits-by-State,pdf.

Witkiewitz, K., et al., 2018. Opioid misuse as a predictor of alcohol treatment outcomes in the COMBINE study: mediation by medication adherence. Alcohol. Clin. Exp. Res. 42.

Wolfers, T., et al., 2018. Brain mapping takes next step toward precision psychiatry. JAMA Psychiatry. https://doi.org/10.1001/jamapsychiatry.2018.2467.

Section 2: Urine Testing

American Society of Addiction Medicine, 2017. Appropriate use of drug testing in clinical addiction medicine, consensus statement. J. Addict. Med. 11 (3).

Baselt, R.C., 2011. Disposition of Toxic Drugs and Chemicals in Man. Biomedical Publications.

Controlled Substance Monitoring and Drugs of Abuse Testing, 2014. http://medicare.fsco.com/Fee Lookup/LCDDisplay.asp?id=DL35654&submitcode=+Sub.

Jarvis, M., et al., 2017. Appropriate use of drug testing in clinical addiction medicine. J Addict. Med. 11, 163.

Kirsh, K.L., Baxter, L.E., et al., 2015. A survey of members' knowledge, attitudes, and practices in urine drug testing. J. Addict. Med. 9, 399.

Laboratory Director Responsibilities, 2014. Cola's Insights. www.Cola.org.

Langman, L.J., Jannetto, P.J., 2014. Laboratory medicine practice guidelines: using clinical laboratory tests to monitor drug therapy in pain management patients. Natl. Acad. Clin. Biochem. https://www.aacc.org/~/media/files/ncab Impg sopc jan 2014.pdf?la=en.

Shea, C.L. (Ed.), 2013. Drug Testing: A White Paper of the American Society of Addiction Medicine (ASAM). http://www.ASAM.org.

Urine adulterant test for oxidants yields positive results from microbial-contaminated urine, 2004. J. Anal. Tox. 28.

Section 3: Outpatient Substance Abuse Detoxification and Medication Assisted Therapy (MAT)

Abuse-Deterrent Opioid Formulations. JAMA 314, 1744.

Acevido, A., 2018. Improving quality of care for SUDS: where do we go from here. J. Addict. Med. 12, 257.

Adams, J.M., 2018. Increasing nalaxone awareness and use: the role of health catre practitioners. JAMA 319, 2073.

Alderks, C.E., 2017. Trend in the use of methadone, buprinorphine and extended release naltrexone at substance abuse treatment facilities: 2003–2015. CBHSQ Rep. Center for Behavioral Health, Statistics, and Quality, Substance Abuse and Mental Health Services Administration, Rockville MD.

American Association for the Treatment of Opioid dependence, Inc. http://www.aatod.org/guidelines-for-addressing-benzodiazepine-usin-opioid-treatment-programs-otps/#_edn2?utm_source=Copy+of+2017+Medic.

American Psychiatric Association, 2010. Practice Guideline for the Treatment of Patients with Panic Disorder, second ed. Washington, DC. https://psychiatryonline.org/pb/assest/raw/sitewide/practice_guidelines/guidelines/panicdisorder.pdf.

Ammerman, S., Tau, G.Z., 2016. Weeding out the truth: adolescents and cannabis. J. Addict. Med. 10, 75.

Ammerman, S., Tau, G.Z., Casperson, 2016. Weeding out the truth: adolescents and cannabis: case and discussion. J. Addict. Med. 10, 83.

Azofeifa, A., Mattson, M., Grant, A., 2016. Monitoring marijuana use in the United States. JAMA 316, 1765.

Baggish, A.L., et al., 2017. Cardiovascular toxicity of illicit anabolic-androgenic steroid use. Circulation. https://doi.org/10.1161/CIRCULATIONAHA.116.026945.

Bagnardi, V., Rota, M., et al., 2015. Alcohol consumption and site-specific cancer risk: a comprehensive dose-response meta analysis. Br. J. Cancer 112, 580.

Baumann, M.H., Partilla, J.S., et al., 2012. Powerful cocaine-like actions of 3,4-mthylenedioxypyrovalerone (MDPV),A principal constituent of psychoactive "bath salts" products. Neuropsychopharmcology. https://doi.org/10.1038/npp.2012.204.

Belkin, et al., 2017. Ameliorative response to detoxification, psychotherapy, and medical management in patients maintained on opioids for pain. Am. J. Addict. https://doi.org/10.1111/ajad.12605. PMID: 28800186.

Bensley, K.M., et al., 2018. Posttraumatic stress disorder symptom association with subsequent risky and problem drinking initiation. J. Addict. Med. 12, 353.

Bentinger, M., et al., 2010. Co-enzyme CoQ-10. Biosynthesis and functions. Biochem. Biophysical Res. Commun. 396, 74.

Bradford, A.C., et al., 2018. JAMA Int. Med. https://doi.org/10.1001/jamainternmed.2018.0266.

Burish, M., 2018. Treatment of Kratom dependence with buprinorphine-naloxone maintenance. J. Addict. Med. 12, 481.

Burns, Z.A., et al., 2018. Cannabis addiction and the brain: a review. J. Neuroimmune Pharmacol. https://doi.org/10.1007/s11481-018-97820g.

Centers for Disease Control and Prevention: Opioid Overdose, 2017. www.cdc.gov/drugoverdose/data/statedeaths.html.

Clinical Institute Withdrawal Assessment for Alcohol (CIWA-Ar) Scale, 1991. J. Clin. Psychopharmacol. 11, 291.

Cunningham, C., Fishman, M. (consultants). The ASAM National Practice Guidelines for the Use of Medications in the Treatment of Addiction Involving Opioid Use. http://

www.asam.org/docs/default-source/practice-support/ guidelines-and-consensus-docs/national-practice guide-lines.pdf.

Daley, J., 2018. Ensuring timely access to quality care for US veterans. JAMA 319, 439.

DEA, 2017 DEA- A Briefing Guide for First Responders-Fentanyl and Fentanyl Analogues. www.dea.gov, www.cdc.gov/drugoverdose/opioids/fentanyl.html.

Dedge, M., 2017. Link between intestinal fungi and alcoholic liver disease grows stronger: a recent study provides evidence to the support the correlation of alcoholic liver disease and bacterial overgrowth in the intestines. http://www.mdedge.com/fedprac/ARTICLE/142748/ADDICTION-MEDICINE/LINK-BETWEEN-INTESTINAL-FUNGI-AND ALCOHOLIC LIVER-DISEASE?UTM_SOURCE=clin_p.

Di Forti, M., et al., 2013. Daily use, especially of high potency cannabis, drives the earlier onset of psychosis in cannabis users. Schizophr. Bull. 40, 1509.

Dowell, D., et al., 2017. Underlying factors in drug overdose deaths. J. Am. Med. Assoc. 318, 2295.

Drug Facts, 2012. Synthetic Cathinones ("Bath Salts"). National Institute on Drug Abuse. http://www.drugabuse.gov/publications/drugfacts/synthetic-cathinones-bath-salts.

Dunn, K.F., Saulsgiver, K.A., et al., 2015. Characterizing opioid withdrawal during double-blind buprinorphine detoxification. Drug Alcohol Depend. http://www.drugqnd alcoholdependence.com/article/S0376-8716(15)00135-0/abstract?rss=yes.

Elkashef, A., Kahn, R., et al., 2012. Topiramine for the treatment of methamphatamine addiction: a multi-center placebo-controlled trial. Addiction 107, 1297.

Enoch, M.A., Hodgkinson, C.A., 2016. GABBR1 and SLC6A1, two genes involved in modulation of GABA synaptic transmission, influence risk for alcoholism: results from three ethnically diverse populations. Alcohol. Clin. Exp. Res. 40, 93. http://onlinelibrary.wiley.com/doi/10.111/acer.12929/full.

FDA, 2017. Safe to Prescribe Benzodiazepines to Patients Being Treated for Opioid Addiction. https://www.fda.gov/Safety/MedWatch/SafetyInformation/SafetyAlertsforHumanMedicalProducts/ucm5elqTrackld=e65014b0f99945b087eaca49bf2c9d77&elq=828600127eb142189c384795e42d0def&elqaid=531&e.

FDA and Kratom, 2017. News Events/Newsroom/Press. Announcements/ucm584970.htm.

FDA Issues Class-wide Labeling Changes for Testosterone, Other Anabolic Steroids, 2016. www.fda.gov/Drugs/DrugSafety/ucm526206.htm.

FDA Approves First Once-Monthly Buprenorphine Injection, A Medication-Assisted Treatment Option for Opioid Use Disorder, 2017. FDA. www.fda.gov/NewsEvents/Newsroom/PressAnnouncements/ucm587312.htm?utm_campaign=11302017_PR_FDA%20bunep&utm_medium=email&utm_source=Eloqua.

FDA Approves the First Non-opioid Treatment for Management of Opioid Withdrawal Symptoms in Adults 5/16/18.

Fentanyl Patch Dosage Determination, 2008. Ortho-McNeill. http://www.globalrph.com/fentconv.htm.

Filip, M., et al., 2015. GABAB receptor as therapeutic strategy in substance abuse disorders: focus on positive allosteric modulators. Neuropharmacology 88, 36.

Frank, J.W., et al., 2017. Patient outcomes in dose reduction or discontinuation of long-term opiate therapy: a systematic review. Ann. Intern. Med. 167, 181.

Freeman, C.R., et al., 2018. Emotional recognition biases in alcohol use disorder. Alcohol. Clin. Exp. Res. https://doi.org/10.1111/acer.13802.

Furukawa, T.A., et al., 2016. Comparative efficacy and acceptability of first generation and second generation antidepressants in the acute treatment of major depression: protocol for a network analysis. BMJ Open e010909. https://doi.org/10.1136/bmjopen-2015-010919.

Gomes, T., et al., 2018. Pregabalin and the risk for opioid-related death: a nested case-control study. Ann. Intern. Med. https://doi.org/10.7326/M18-1136.

Gopalakrishna, G., Oluwole, P., et al., Two case reports on use of prazosin for drug dreams. J. Addict. Med. 10, 129.

Gorelick, D.A., 2012. Pharmacokinetic strategies for treatment of drug overdose and addiction. Future Med. Chem. 4, 227.

Gottlieb, S., 2017. Support for treating opioid addiction with medication. J. Am. Med. Assoc. 318, 2071.

Griffin, E.A., et al., 2017. Prior alcohol use enhances vulnerability to compulsive cocaine self-administration by promoting degradation of HDAC4 and HDAC5. Sci. Adv. 3 (11), e1701682. https://doi.org/10.1126/sciadv.1701682.

Hill, K.P., 2017. Cannabis use and risk for substance use disorders and mood and anxiety disorders. JAMA 317, 1070.

Hogue, A., et al., 2014. Evidenced base on outpatient behavioral treatments for adolescent substance use:updates and recommendations 2007−2013. J. Clin. Child. Adol. Psychol. 43, 695.

Jansson, L.M., et al., 2018. Perinatal marijuana use and the developing child. JAMA 320, 545.

Johansen, P.O., Krebs, T.S., 2015. Psychodelics not linked to mental health problems or suicidal behavior: a population study. J. Psychopharmacol. 29, 270.

Kamal, R.M., Dijkstra, B.A., et al., 2016. The effect of co-occurring substance use on gamma-hydrobutyric acid withdrawal syndrome. J. Addict. Med. 10, 229.

Kampman, K., et al., 2015. ASAM Quality Improvement Council the ASAM National Practice Guidelines for the Use of Medications in the Treatment of Addiction Involving Opioid Use. www.asam.org/docs/defsault-source/practice-support/guidelines-and-consensus-docs/asam-national-practice-guideline-suppliment.pdf.

Kanny, D., et al., 2018. Total binge drinks consumed by US adults 2015. Am. J. Prev. Med. 54, 486.

Konghom, S., Verachai, V., et al., 2010. Treatment for inhalant dependence and abuse. Cochrane Database Syst. Rev. (12), CD007537.

Kranzler, H.R., Soyka, M., 2018. Diagnosis and pharmacotherapy of alcohol use disorder: a review. JAMA 320, 815.

Kravitz, R.L., 2017. Direct-to-consumer advertising of androgen replacement therapy. JAMA 317, 1124.

Krebs, E.E., 2018. Effect of opioid vs. non-opioid medications on pain-related function in patients with chronic back pain or hip or knee osteoarthritis pain: the SPACE randomized clinical trial. JAMA 319, 872.

Kroenke, K., Cheville, A., 2017. Management of chronic pain in the aftermath of the opioid backlash. JAMA 317, 2365.

Layton, J.B., et al., 2017. Association between direct-to-consumer advertising and testosterone testing and initiation in the United States, 2009–2013. JAMA 317, 1159.

Lingford-Hughes, A.R., et al., 2012. BAP updated guidelines, evidence based guidelines for the pharmacological management of substance abuse, harmful use, addiction and comorbidity: recommendations from BAP. J. Psychopharmacol. 26, 899.

Lopez, G., 2017. There is a Highly Successful Treatment for Opioid Addiction. But Stigma is Holding it Back. www.vox.com/science-and-health/2017/7/20/15937896/medication-assisted-treatment-methadone-buprinorphine-naltrexone.

Low Dose Protocol for the Use of Buprinorphine and Suboxone, 2010. Ohio Department of Health.

Lubarski, K., Odom, A., et al., 2014. Understanding the dangers of synthetic cannabinoids. J. Addict. Med. https://doi.org/10.97/ADM.000000000040.

Marder, J., 2012. Bath Salts: The Drug that Never Lets Go. http://www.pbs.org/newshour/topics.

Martin, S.A., et al., 2018. The next stage of buprinorphine care for opioid use disorder. Ann. Intern. Med. https://doi.org/10.7326/M18-1625.

Martinez, D., Trifilieff, P., 2015a. A Review of Potential Pharmacological Treatments for Cannabis Abuse. ASAM Magazine. http://www.asam.org/magazine/read/article/2015/04/13.

Martinez, D., Trifilieff, P., 2015b. Repurposing Medications to Treat Addiction. ASAM Magazine. http://www.asam.org/magazine/read/article/2015/12/13/repurposing -medications-to-treat-addiction?utm_medium=email&utm_campaign=ASA.

Morley, K.C., Baillie, A., et al., 2014. Baclofen for the treatment of alcohol dependence and possible role of comorbid anxiety. Alcohol Alcohol. https://doi.org/10.1093/alcalc/agu062.

Nacca, N., Vatti, D., et al., 2013. The synthetic cannabinoid withdrawal syndrome. J. Addict. Med. 7, 296.

National Practice Guidelines for Medications for the Treatment of Opioid Use Disorder, 2015. www.ASAM.org.

Nielsen, S., et al., 2017. Opioid agonist treatment for patients with dependence on prescription opioids. JAMA 317, 967.

Parran, T.V., Adelman, C.A., et al., 2009. Long-Term outcomes of office-based buprinorphine/nalaxone maintenance therapy. Drug Alcohol Depend. https://doi.org/10.1016/j.drugalcdep.2009.07.013.

Pope, H.C., et al., 2017. Body image disorders and abuse of anabolic-androgenic steroids among men. JAMA 317, 23.

Prazocin and Doxazocin for PTSD are underutilized and underdosed, 2017. Curr. Psychiatry 16, 19.

Prekupec, M.P., et al., 2017. Misuse of novel synthetic opiates: a deadly new trend. J. Addict. Med. 11, 256.

Ramaekers, J.G., 2018. Driving under the influence of Cannabis: an increasing public health concern. JAMA 319, 1433.

Rao, R.B., Nelson, L.S., 2017. The new opioid epidemic: prescriptions, synthetics, and street drugs. Emerg. Med. 49, 64.

Ray, L.A., Bujarski, S., et al., 2015. The effect of naltrexone on subjective response to methamphetamine in a clinical sample: a double blind, placebo controlled laboratory study. Neuropsych. Pharm. https://doi.org/10.1038/npp.2015.83.

Rege, S.V., et al., 2018. Rends and characteristics of nalaxone therapy reported to U.S. poison centers. Addiction. https://doi.org/10.1111/add.14378.

Robinson, S., Meeks, Geniza, C., 2014. Medication for alcohol use disorders: which agents work best? Curr. Psychiatry 13, 22.

Saitz, R., 2017. Should benzodiazepines be used to treat anxiety in people with substance abuse disorders? Contentious debate with similar conclusions. J. Addict. Med. 11, 83.

SAMSHA-HHS, 2012. Opioid drugs in maintenance and detoxification treatment of opiate addiction: proposed modification of dispensing restrictions for buprinorphine and buprinorphine combination as used in approved opioid treatment medications. Federal Reg. 77, 72752.

Scharfstein, J.M., 2018. A new year's wish on opioids. JAMA 319, 537.

Schneiderhan, J., et al., 2017. Primary care of patients with chronic pain. JAMA 317, 2367.

Shoptaw, S.J., Kao, U., et al., 2009. Treatment for amphetamine withdrawal. Cochrane Database Syst. Rev. (2), CD003021.

Sidney, S., et al., 2018. Comparative trends in heart disease,stroke, all cause mortality in the United States and a large integrated health care system. Am. J. Med. 131, 829.

Smith, D.J., et al., 2017. Transforming the military health system. J. Am. Med. Assoc. 318, 2427.

Sofouglu, M., Rosenheck, R., Petrakis, 2014. Pharmacological treatment of co-morbid PTSD and substance use disorder: recent progress. Addict. Behav. 30, 428.

Srivastava, A.B., Gold, M.S., 2017. Co-occurring disorders-substance use disorder and depression. Dir. Psychiatry 37, 77.

Stassinos, G.L., Klein-Schwartz, W., 2016. Bupropion "abuse" reported to US poison centers. J. Addict. Med. 10, 357.

Stopops, W.W., 2014. Combination pharmacotherapies for stimulant use disorder: a review of clinical findings and recommendation for future research. Expert Rev. Clin. Pharm. 7, 363.

Sun, E.C., et al., 2017. Association between concurrent use of prescription opioids and benzodiazepines and overdose: retrospective analysis. BMJ. https://doi.org/10.1136/vmj.j760.

Talih, F., Fattal, O., Malone, D., 2007. Anabolic steroid abuse: psychiatric and physical costs. Clevel Clinic. J. Med. 74, 341.

Tawakol, A., et al., 2017. Relation between resting amygdalar activity and cardiovascular events: a longitudinal and cohort study. Lancet 389 (10071), 834–885. https://doi.org/10.1016/S0140-6736(16)6731714-7.

Terry-McElrath, Y.M., et al., 2014. Energy drinks, soft drinks, and substance use among United States secondary school students. J. Addict. Med. 8, 6.

The ASAM National Practice guideline for the use of medications in the treatment of addiction involving opioid use, 2015. J. Addict. Med. 9 (1). www.ASAM.org.

The ASAM Performance Measures for the Addiction Specialist Physician, 2014. www.ASAM.org.

The US Department of Health and Human Services Guide to Comprehensive Drug Treatment or Detoxification, 2006.

Tsai, J., Shen, J., 2017. Exploring the link between post-traumatic stress disorder and inflammation related medical conditions: an epidemiological examination. Psychiatr Q. 88, 909.

US Preventive Task Force Recommendation Statement: screening and behavioral counseling interventions to reduce unhealthy alcohol use in adolescents and adults, 2018. JAMA 320, 1899.

Vatsalva, V., Gowin, J.L., et al., 2015. Effects of varenicline on neural correlates of alcohol salience in heavy drinkers. Int. J. Neuropsychopharm. https://doi.org/10.1093/ijnp/pyv068.

Vilakshan, A., et al., 2018. The emerging role of inhaled heroin in the opioid epidemic. JAMA Neurol. https://doi.org/10.10001/jamaneurol.2018.1693.

Von Theobald, et al., 2017. Inpatient gamma-hydroxtbyurate detoxification: a case report describing day to day therapeutic management. J. Addict. Med. 11, 231.

Wachman, E.F., et al., 2018. Neonatal abstinence syndrome. JAMA 319, 1363.

Wale, R., et al., 2010. Fatty acids from fish: the anti-inflammatory potential of long chain omega 3 fatty acids. Nutr. Rev. 68, 280.

Wasantha Parakrama, J., Ahmed Hassan, Y.A., 2014. Multiple and substitute addictions involving prescription drugs misuse among 12th graders: gateway theory revisited with market basket analysis. J. Addict. Med. https://doi.org/10.1097/ADM0000000000000012.

Weinberger, A.H., et al., 2018. Is cannibis use associated with increased risk of cigarette smoking initiation, persistence, and relapse. J. Clin. Psychiat. https://doi.org/10.4088/JCP.17m11522.

Wesson, D.R., Ling, W., 2003. The clinical opioid withdrawal scale (COWS). J. Psychoactive Drugs 35, 253.

Wiffin, P.J., et al., 2017. Gabapentin for chronic neuropathic pain in adults. Cochrane Database Syst. Rev. 6, CD007928. https://doi.org/10.1002/14651858.CD007938.pub4. PMID: 2859747.

Wong, J., et al., 2018. Does maternal buprinorphine dose affect severity or incidence of neonatal abstinence syndrome. J. Addict. Med. 12, 435.

Wood, A.M., et al., 2018. Risk thresholds for alcohol consumption: combined analysis of individual-participant data for 599912 current drinkers in 83 prospective studies. Lancet 391, 1513.

Wu, H., et al., 2017. Closing the loop on impulsivity via nucleus accumbens delta band Activity in mice and man. Proc. Natl. Acad. Sci. U.S.A. https://doi.org/10.1073/pnas.171214114 pii:2017/12214.

Yamamomoto, T., Friedman, S.E., 2017. Torsades de Pointes in severe alcohol withdrawal and cirrhosis: implications for risk stratification and monitoring: close monitoring of the QT interval and aggressive management of withdrawal, repletion of electrolytes, and telemetry monitoring may prevent life-threatening arrhythmias for patients being treated for acute alcohol withdrawal. Fed. Pract. 34, 38.

Yarborough, B.H., et al., 2018. Patient and system characteristics associated with performance on the HEDIS measures of alcohol and drug treatment initiation and engagement. J. Addict. Med. 12, 278.

Zaleska-Kaszubska, J., 2015. Is immunotherapy an opportunity for effective treatment of drug addiction. Vaccine 33, 6545.

Zhang, Y., et al., 2016. Inhibition of lactate transport erases drug memory and prevents drug relapse. Biol. Psychiat. 79, 928.

Zhao, R.J., Lin, S.H., et al., 2016. Probing of serotonin transporter availability among male cigarette smokers: a SPECT study with 123I ADAM. J. Addict. Med. 10, 89.

Section 4: Smoking Cessation Protocol

Baker, T.B., et al., 2016. Effects of nicotine patch vs combination nicotine replacement therapy on smoking cessation at 26 weeks: a randomized clinical trial. JAMA 315, 371.

Breakthrough in Mapping Nicotine Addiction Could Help Researchers Improve Treatment, 2016. UT Southwest Medical Center. https://www.sciencedaily.com/releases/2016/10/161003120207.htm.

Brennan, T.A., Schroeder, 2014. Ending sales of tobacco products in pharmacies. JAMA. https://doi.org/10.100/jama.2014.686.

Cawley, J., Dragone, D., Von Hinkle Kessler Scholder, S., 2016. The demand for cigarettes as derived from the demand for weight loss: a theoretical and empirical investigation. Health Econ. 25, 8.

Chang, J.S., Chiang, C.H., et al., 2015. Combination therapy of varencicline with nicotine replacement therapy is better than varencicline alone: a systematic review and meta-analysis of randomized controlled trials. BMC Public Health 15, 689.

Chang, P.Y., et al., 2016. Comparative effectiveness of smoking cessation medications: a national prospective cohort from Taiwan. PLoS One 11 (11), e0166992. PMID: 27893843.

Dai, H., et al., 2018. Electronic cigarettes and future marijuana use: a longitudinal study. Pediatrics 141, e20173787.

Dietz, W.H., Douglas, J.D., Brownson, R.C., 2016. Tobacco avoidance, physical activity, and nutrition for a healthy start. JAMA 316, 1645.

FDA Drug Safety Communication: FDA Warning for Stop Smoking Drug Chantix (Varencicline) to Include Potential Alcohol Interaction, Rare Seizures, and Studies of Side Effects on Neuropshyciatric Behavior or Thinking, 2015. http://www.fda.gov/Drugs/DrugSafety/ucm436494.htm.

FDA's Youth Prevention Plan, 2018. https://www.fda.gov//TobaccoProducts/PublicHealthEducation/ProtectingKidsfromTobacco/ucm608433.htm.

Gaznick, N.V., Anthenelli, R.M., 2017. E-cigarettes and vapes: do they work for smoking cessation and should we be recommending their use. Curr. Psychiatry 16, 30.

Hartman-Boyce, J., McRobbie, H., et al., 2016. Electronic cigarettes for smoking cessation. Cochrane Database Syst. Rev. 9 https://doi.org/10.1002/14651858.CD010216.pub3. PMID: 27622384.

Hatsukami, D.K., et al., 2018. Effect of immediate vs gradual reduction in nicotine content of cigarettes on biomarkers of smoke exposure: a randomized clinical trial. JAMA 320, 880.

Kandel, E.R., Kandel, D.B., 2014. A molecular basis for nicotine as a gateway drug. N. Engl. J. Med. 371, 932.

King, A.C., Cao, D., et al., 2013. Naltrexone reduction of long-term smoking cessation weight gain in women but not in men: a randomized controlled trial. Biol. Psychiat. 73, 924.

Leventhal, A.M., Stone, M.D., et al., 2016. Association of e-cigarette vaping and progression to heavier patterns of cigarette smoking. JAMA 316, 1918.

Richman, I., Krumholtz, H.M., 2018. Lessons from the opioid epidemic to reinvigorate tobacco control activities. JAMA 319, 399.

Richtel, M., 2014. Selling a Poison by the Barrel: Liquid Nicotine for E-Cigarettes. The New York Times.

Rubin, R., 2017. Will the FDA's new tobacco strategy be a game changer? J. Am. Med. Assoc. 318, 2413.

Selya, A., et al., 2018. Evaluating the mutual pathways among electronic cigarette use, conventional smoking and nicotine dependence. Addiction 113 (2), 325−333.

Shahab, L., et al., 2017. Nicotine, carcinogen, and toxin exposure in long-term e-cigarette and nicotine replacement therapy users: a cross sectional study. Ann. Intern. Med. https://doi.org/10.7326/M16-1107. PMID: 28166548.

Sheikhattari, P., Apata, J., et al., 2016. Examining smoking cessation in a community-based versus clinic-based participatory research. J. Community Health. https://doi.org/10.1007/s10900-16-0264-9. PMID: 27688221.

Substance Abuse and Mental Health Services Administration: National Survey on Drug Use and Health (NSDUH) 2008−2015, 2015. https://www.samsha.gov/samsha-data-outcomes-quality/major-data-collections/reports-detailed-tables-2015-NSDUH.

Substance Abuse and Mental Health Services Administration (SAMSHA), 2018. Implementing Tobacco Cessation Programs in Substance Abuse Disorder Treatment Settings: A Quick Guide for Program Directors and Clinicians. HHS Publication No. SMA 18-5069QG.

Tseng, T.Y., et al., 2016. A randomized trial comparing the effect of nicotine versus placebo electronic cigarettes on smoking reduction among young adult smokers. Nicotine Tob. Res. pii: ntw071.

Weaver, M., Breland, A., et al., 2014. Electronic cigarettes: a review of safety and clinical issues. J. Addict. Med. 8, 234.

Williams, J.M., Steinberg, M.L., et al., 2016. An argument for change in tobacco treatment options guided by the ASAM criteria for patient placement. J. Addict. Med. 10, 291.

Zhu, H., Wu, L.T., Trends and correlates of cannabis-involved emergency department visits: 2001−2011. J. Addict. Med. 10, 429.

Section 5: Long Term Substance Cessation Medications

Agabiuo, R., Preti, A., Gessa, G.L., 2013. Efficacy and tolerability of baclofen in substance use disorders: a systematic review. Eur. Addict. Res. 19, 325.

Amato, L., Minozzi, S., et al., 2011. Dopamine antagonists for the treatment of cocaine dependence. Cochrane Database Syst. Rev. 12, CD003352.

Carpenter, J.E., et al., 2018. An overview of pharmacotherapy options for alcohol use disorder. Fed. Pract. 35, 48.

Clinical Use of Extended-Release Inject Able Naltrexone in the Treatment of Opioid Use Disorder: A Brief Guide, 2015. SAMHSA HHS Publication No.(SMA) 14-4892, Rockville MD.

Johnson, B.A., Ait Daoud, N., 2010. Topiramate in the new generation of drugs: efficacy in treatment of alcoholic patients. Curr. Pharm. Des. 16, 2103.

Kampman, K.M., 2005. New medications for the treatment of cocaine dependence. Psychiatry 2, 44.

Karila, L., Gorelick, D., et al., 2008. New treatments for cocaine dependence: a focused review. Int. J. Neuropharmacol. 11, 425.

Krampe, H., Stewicki, S., et al., 2006. Follow up of 180 alcoholic patients of up to seven years after outpatient treatment: impact of alcohol deterrents on outcome. Alcohol. Clin. Exp. Res. 30, 86.

Kranzler, H.R., Soyka, M., 2018. Diagnosis and pharmacotherapy of alcohol use disorder: a review. JAMA 320, 815.

Leggio, L., Garbutt, J.C., Addolorato, G., 2010. Effectiveness and safety of baclofen in the treatment of alcohol dependent patients. CNS Neurol. Disord. Drug Targets 9, 33.

Liu, J., Wang, L.N., 2015. Baclofen for alcohol withdrawal. Cochrane Database Syst. Rev. 4, CD008502. https://doi.org/10.1002/14651858.CD008502.pub4. PMID: 25836263.

Lyon, J., 2017. More treatments on deck for alcohol use disorder. JAMA 317, 2267.

Mirijello, A., et al., 2015. GABA-B agonists for treatment of alcohol use disorder. Curr. Pharm. Des. 21, 3367.

Neural Mechanisms Underlying Drug Cravings, 2013. Science Daily. http://www.sciencedaily.com/releases/2013/01/130128151914.htm.

Olsen, Y., Scharfstein, J.M., 2014. Confronting the stigma of opioid use disorder-and its treatment. JAMA. https://doi.org/10.100/JAMA.2014.2147.

Oral naltrexone as maintenance treatment to prevent relapse in opioid addicts who have undergone detoxification, 2011. Cochrane Database Syst. Rev. http://www.ncbi.nih.gov/pubmedhealth/PMH0010991.

O'Malley, S.S., et al., 2017. Effect of Varenicline combined with medical management of alcohol use disorder with comorbid smoking: a randomized clinical trial. JAMA Psychiatry. https://doi.org/10.1002/jamapsychiatry.2017.3544.

Reus, V.I., et al., 2018. APA guideline backs naltrexone, acomprasate for alcohol use disorder. Am. J. Psychiatry 175, 86.

Schurks, M., Overlack, M., Bonnet, U., 2005. Naltrexone treatment of combined alcohol and opioid dependence: deterioration of Co-morbid major depression. Pharmacopsychiatry 38, 100.

Setawian, E., Cox, S.M., et al., 2011. The effect of naltrexone on alcohol's stimulant properties and self-administration behavior in social drinkers: influence of gender and genotype. Alcohol. Clin. Exp. Res. 35, 1134.

Singal, A.K., et al., 2018. Guidelines for alcohol withdrawal treatment in advanced liver disease. Am. J. Gastroenterol. https://doi.org/10.1038/ajg.2017.469.

Sullivan, M.A., et al., 2018. XR –naltrexone beats oral medication for opioid use disorder. Am. J. Psychiatry. https://doi.org/10.1176/appi.ajp.2018.17070732.

Vivitrol (Prescribing Information), 2013. Alkermes Inc. Rev, Waltham MA.

Section 6: Common Substance Abuse Associated Sexually Transmitted Diseases

Abara, W.E., et al., 2017. Hepatitis B vaccination, screening, and linkage to care: best practice advice from the American College of Physicians and Centers for Disease Control and Prevention. Ann. Intern. Med. 167, 794.

Ahmed, O., et al., 2018. NASH rapidly overtaking hepatitis C as a cause of liver cancer. J. Clin. Exp. Hepatol. https://doi.org/10.1016/j.jceh.2018.02.006.

Bersoff-Matcha, S.J., et al., 2017. Hepatitis B virus reactivation associated with direct-acting antiviral therapy for chronic hepatitis C virus: a review of cases reported to the US food and drug administration adverse events reporting system. Ann. Intern. Med. https://doi.org/10.7326/M17-0377. PMID: 28437794.

Burger, E.A., et al., 2017. Age of acquiring causal human papillomavirus (HPV) infections: leveraging simulation models to explore the natural history of HPV-induced cervical cancer. Clin. Infect. Dis. https://doi.org/10.1093/cid/cix475. PMID: 28531261.

Carrieri, M.P., et al., 2017. Protective effect of coffee consumption on all-cause mortality of French HIV/HCV co-infected patients. J. Hepatol. https://doi.org/10.1016/j.jhep.2017.08.005. PMID: 28942916.

CDC, 2013. A Guide to Comprehensive Hepatitis C Counseling and Testing. cdcinfo@cdc.gov.

CDC. Sexually Transmitted Diseases. https://www.cdc.gov/ncchhstp/atlas.

CDC TB. Guidelines and Recommendations/National. https://npin.cdc.gov/pages/cdc-tb-guidelines-and-recommendations.

Danelishvili, L., et al., 2017. *Mycobacterium tuberculosis* proteome response to anti-tuberculosis compounds reveals metabolic "escape" pathways that prolong bacterial survival. Antimicrob. Agents Chemother. 61 (6) https://doi.org/10.1128/AAC.00430-17.

Dilley, S., et al., 2017. Preventing human pappilomavirus-related cancers: we are all in this together. Am. J. Obstret. Gynecol. 216, 576.

FDA Approved Class Labeling Revisions Regarding the Risk of Hepatitis B Virus Reactivation in Patients Coinfected with Hepatitis C Virus (HCV) and Hepatitis B Virus (HBV, 2017. https://content.govdelivery.com/accounts/USFDA/bullns/18741e2.

Hall, E., et al., 2018. Estimates of state-level chronic hepatitis-C virus infection, stratified by race and sex, United States, 2010. BMC Infect. Dis. https://doi.org/10.1186/s12879-018-3133-6.

Jin, J., 2016. Screening for genital herpes. JAMA 316, 2560.

Jin, J., 2018. HPV infection and Cancer. JAMA 319, 1058.

Kim, D.K., et al., 2017. Advisory Committee on Immunization Practices recommended immunization schedule for adults aged 19 years or older. MMWR Morb. Mortal. Wkly. Rep. 66, 136.

Levy, B.S., 2017. It is time for HPV vaccination to be considered part of routine preventive healthcare. OBG Manag. 29, 17.

Lewinsohn, D.M., et al., 2017. American Thoracic Society, Infectious Disease Society of America and CDC Clinical Practice Guidelines-TB testing for those not likely to be infected. Clin. Infect. Dis. 64, 1.

McQuillin G et al. Prevalence of HPV in Adults Aged 18–69: United States 2011–2014 4/6/17. NCHS Data Brief No. 280.

Moore, M.S., et al., 2018. Effect of hepatocellular carcinoma on mortality among individuals with hepatitis B or C infection in New York City, 2001–2012. Open Forum Infect. Dis. https://doi.org/10.1093/ofid/ofy144.q.

Rubin, R., 2018. Nearly 15% of US HIV infections under diagnosed in 2015. JAMA 319, 114.

Shaffer, M., Ahuja, D., 2017. Hepatitis C: screening changes, treatment advance. J. Fam. Pract. 66, 136.

Tang, L.S.Y., et al., 2018. Chronic hepatitis B infection. JAMA 319, 1802.

Trichomoniasis-CDC Fact Sheet, 2015. http://www.cdc.gov/std/trichomonas/stdfact-trichomoniasis.htm.

Index

Note: Page numbers followed by "f" indicate figures.

Printed and bound by CPI Group (UK) Ltd, Croydon, CR0 4YY

03/10/2024

01040300-0015